Copernicus Books

Sparking Curiosity and Explaining the World

Drawing inspiration from their Renaissance namesake, Copernicus books revolve around scientific curiosity and discovery. Authored by experts from around the world, our books strive to break down barriers and make scientific knowledge more accessible to the public, tackling modern concepts and technologies in a nontechnical and engaging way. Copernicus books are always written with the lay reader in mind, offering introductory forays into different fields to show how the world of science is transforming our daily lives. From astronomy to medicine, business to biology, you will find herein an enriching collection of literature that answers your questions and inspires you to ask even more.

Marcelo Leite

The Psychedelic Science of the Jurema Tree

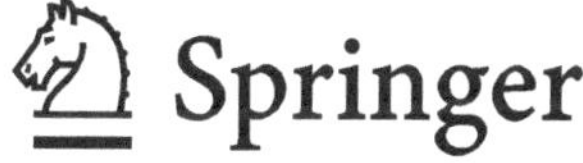 Springer

Marcelo Leite
São Paulo, São Paulo, Brazil

ISSN 2731-8982   ISSN 2731-8990   (electronic)
Copernicus Books
ISBN 978-3-032-22704-1   ISBN 978-3-032-22705-8   (eBook)
https://doi.org/10.1007/978-3-032-22705-8

The original submitted manuscript has been translated into English. The translation was done using artificial intelligence. A subsequent revision was performed by the author(s) to further refine the work and to ensure that the translation is appropriate concerning content and scientific correctness. It may, however, read stylistically different from a conventional translation.

This Springer imprint is published by the registered company Springer Nature Switzerland AG
The registered company address is: Gewerbestrasse 11, 6330 Cham, Switzerland

If disposing of this product, please recycle the paper.

Preface

The fascination with Jurema Sagrada that gave rise to this book began in the final days of 2021, with a visit from Dráulio Barros de Araújo, from the Brain Institute at the Federal University of Rio Grande do Norte (ICEUFRN), to São Paulo. He had previously featured as one of the main figures in my previous book *Psiconautas: Viagens com a ciência psicodélica brasileira* (Fósforo, 2021), alongside Luís Fernando Tófoli, Sidarta Ribeiro, and Stevens "Bitty" Rehen. This quartet of neuroscientist had accompanied me since 2017, when, during my journey through the turbulent waters of the resurgent research on consciousness-altering substances, we met at the Psychedelic Science conference in Oakland, California, and I discovered the submerged continent of clinical studies with MDMA (ecstasy) and psilocybin (from "magic" mushrooms) for psychiatric disorders such as post-traumatic stress and depression.

At the time, this new subject rekindled my enthusiasm for science journalism, after three decades of frustration with the course of climate change and the destruction of the Amazon rainforest. The researcher from UFRN had previously led a pioneering clinical trial to treat depression with ayahuasca, the Amazonian brew containing the psychedelic N,N - dimethyltryptamine (DMT), one of the highlights in *Psiconautas*.

With Araújo's visit, a reporter's curiosity provided a break among the post-pandemic anxieties, opening up a way to the chants and enchantments of Brazil's northeastern backlands: a little-known plant, with deep psychedelic roots in the culture of the original peoples of the caatinga, who rose up with their ancestors and other enslaved people against colonial domination. The scientist explained, during his brief stop in São Paulo, that he was still studying the substance for the same disorder, but now inhaled, purified, and extracted from jurema-preta (black jurema, known by botanists as *Mimosa tenuiflora*), a small tree of the semi-arid region that he collected every month on a farm five hundred kilometers from Natal, the capital of Rio Grande do Norte. He was determined to unravel the function of the compound in the plant, beyond its therapeutic potential in humans. He mentioned in passing that the DMT from jurema had also given rise, under the name nigerine, to an obscure episode in the Brazilian history of science: it was first isolated by a chemist from the state of Pernambuco in the 1940s, intrigued by the powers attributed to the plant by Indigenous people of the backlands who used a beverage prepared from it in rituals—a "wine" from which the psychoactive compound was extracted.

These were the ideal ingredients to tell a story as interesting and important as few others, an undertaking that would have a significant impact on my worldview. I had only heard of black jurema once, from the mouth of a psychonaut present at the first session in which I took ayahuasca, and, in my excitement as a novice, I paid it no mind. Of the ethnic resurgence of peoples in the Northeast, I knew only superficially the story of the Pataxó of Bahia and their struggle for recognition of their traditional territory; as is typical of those from Southeastern Brazil, my attention was focused solely on the Indigenous peoples of the Amazon, and now dozens of peoples from the backlands with a long history of resistance—driven in large part by jurema—were appearing on my radar.

Moreover, the intoxicating rituals had survived and achieved an urban reincarnation, blended with African practices and European magics—first in Catimbó, studied by folklorists Mário de Andrade and Luís da Câmara Cascudo in the first half of the twentieth century, and up to the present day in a religion, Jurema Sagrada (a more recent designation that replaces the earlier, culturally stigmatized term Catimbó, since "catimbozeiro" is almost an insult in various parts of the Northeast), which struggles to escape the shadow of Umbanda, an urban form of Afro-Brazilian religion. Finally, and no less relevant, I realized that the same plant was circulating in neo-shamanic circles and their postmodern blend of mysticisms.

The first steps of this narrative endeavor took shape in three reports for the newspaper *Folha de S. Paulo*, published online in July 2022 in the series "The Resurrection of Jurema." This trio of articles forms the basis of the first chapter of this book, "The Goddess Jurema and the Devil of Science Against the Dragon of Anxiety," which presents the collection of black jurema on

Araújo's family farm, a profile of the researcher and his father, the story of Oswaldo Gonçalves de Lima, the chemist who discovered nigerine/DMT in nature, my participation as a volunteer in the pilot phase of the experiment at the Brain Institute of UFRN with inhaled DMT to treat depression and the efforts of this team to bring the psychedelic substance to Brazil's Unified Health System (SUS).

Next, the book follows the course of my discoveries, in an imperfect chronological order, guided by the mental journey provided by geographic, psychedelic, and philosophical explorations. In the chapter "Origin of Catimbó in Alhandra, former colonial settlement," I recount my trip to the city of Alhandra in the state of Paraíba, considered the epicenter of the religious practice known as Catimbó, which still survives today under the less pejorative name of Jurema Sagrada, persecuted as witchcraft by the Catholic Church, the by the police, and more recently, by evangelical groups. There, my guides in a lay initiation into the religion were the young juremeira Nayanne Alves dos Santos and the spiritualist Dona Raquel, who took me to the little church of Acais, to the memorials of the masters Flósculo and Zezinho, to the Cantinho dos Benzedores, to the Portal da Encantaria, and to the Pedra de Xangô on Tambaba beach. Through them, I also met three generations of Jurema masters—Ciriaco, Nina, and Lucas—who still face harassment from other religious denominations, as well as rivalry between temples and family tragedies; I also learned the stories of legendary female masters such as Maria do Acais and Jardecilha, or Zefinha de Tiíno, and of the fierce struggle to keep the science of Jurema alive in its birthplace.

Although the Catimbó-Jurema tradition surfaced there, it was not in Alhandra that it was formed. Its roots reach much deeper into Brazil's history, with the earliest records of ritual use of jurema beverages dating back to the seventeenth and eighteenth centuries, associated with tobacco fumigations in pipes and chants accompanied by maracás, the gourd rattles ubiquitous among the Indigenous peoples of the Northeast. The quest to understand this Indigenous matrix of the elusive religion, virtually unknown in the rest of the country, motivated further journeys to towns in the backlands and along the northeastern coast. The first stop was in Caruaru, where anthropologist Sandro Guimarães de Salles granted access to dozens of Indigenous education students at the Agreste Academic Center, a campus of the Federal University of Pernambuco in the city famous for its clay figurines. With Salles's help, one of the leading figures in the new wave of anthropological studies on Jurema Sagrada, I made contact with members of the Potiguara people in Baía da Traição and the Fulni-ô in Águas Belas, whose villages and rituals I had the privilege to visit and describe in the third chapter, on Indigenous resistance in the Northeast centered on black jurema. Following the clues and teachings from the books and articles of Salles and scholars such as Rodrigo Grünewald, Luiz Assunção, Dilaine Sampaio, Estêvão Palitot, and Guilherme Medeiros, I delved into the chronicles of uprisings and persecutions driven by the failed attempts of the Catholic Inquisition, the Portuguese Crown, the Brazilian Empire, and the colonial police to suppress the backlands' faith in enchanted beings—masters, caboclos, old Black spirits, exus, pombajiras, and others—which would later merge with the magics of enslaved Africans and expatriated Europeans to expand the pantheon of entities still incorporated by juremeiros in their rituals. I close this chapter with a pale sketch of this religiosity, kept secret for centuries as a way to preserve a core of autonomy in the face of the genocidal onslaught of the invading culture.

In the chapter "Jurema Sagrada at the Crossroads between Catimbó and Umbanda," I grapple with the most obscure question for newcomers to the illuminated terreiros of Jurema: to what extent can one say, or should one not say, that this religion is a form of Umbanda? There was undoubtedly a process of syncretism with African traditions in several waves, the first probably still in colonial times, when enslaved Indigenous and Black people met in Catholic missions and in the mocambos and quilombos of the interior—encounters in which deities, spirits, and ancestors also joined forces to fight a common enemy. In the nineteenth century, Catimbó was influenced by Kardecist spiritism through Umbanda, which, in the following century, would provide shelter—through the institutionalization of Umbanda federations arriving in the Northeast—for Jurema rituals under police repression. These intertwined roots materialized for me at the Casa das Matas do Reis Malunguinho terreiro in Recife, in the form of the enchanted beings Zé Pelintra and Malunguinho, who manifested there, and months later, at the Festa do Amaro in Brejo do Burgo, with Pankararé Indigenous people dancing with the praiás and accompanied by entities such as Caboclo Aboiador and Capitão, whose embraces and messages stirred unknown emotions within me. Among them, reverence for the mysteries—something my rationalism could not then comprehend, but which did not, for that reason, turn me into a believer.

The plant *Mimosa tenuiflora*, on the other hand, had long since left the secrecy of Jurema science in Indigenous and Catimbó terreiros to be embraced by the academic sciences of ethnopharmacology, biomedical research, and associated psychonautics. My guide on this journey, which gave rise to the chapter "Juremahuasca, a sacrament challenging doctrines," was the anthropologist Rodrigo Grünewald, whom I interviewed on two occasions, in Rio de Janeiro, his city of origin, and in Campina Grande, where he lectures at the Federal University of Paraíba. He was among the first ayahuasca practitioners from the Santo Daime and Barquinha churches in Rio de Janeiro to prepare and conduct rituals with a beverage nicknamed juremahuasca, in which black jurema is combined with Syrian rue, a plant native to the arid regions of the Mediterranean, to potentiate the psychedelic effect of DMT contained in the former. Juremahuasca had been proposed as a simplified and inexpensive option for psychonauts worldwide by Jonathan Ott, an American chemist based in Mexico, but it was through Yatra, a Brazilian therapist living in the Netherlands, that Grünewald introduced black jurema into the neo-shamanic circles of the 1990s. Another important popularizer of DMT was the pioneering scientist Rick Strassman, who dubbed it the Spirit Molecule in the title of a famous book, planting in the minds of psychonauts seeds of metaphysical speculation about the pineal gland, the cosmic powers of the substance, and its supposed function as an esoteric antenna in the brain.

The DMT from black jurema also became popular among New Age psychonauts and neo-shamanism enthusiasts in the form of changa—crystals that can be vaporized and smoked, sometimes mixed with herbs. I had the opportunity to try it at an equinox festival on a paradisiacal beach in Bahia, when an explosion of colors and arabesques left me prostrate in the nave of a fantastic mosque, a journey that lasted a few minutes and was similar to the first dose of DMT I inhaled during the Natalexperiment.

In the sixth chapter, "Changa and DMT Crystals, Engines of Cosmopolitan Neo-shamanism," I recount the brief adventure with changa and how a variant of this smoked modality, "aussiewaska," emerged in Australia, where the source of DMT is acacias, trees somewhat related to black jurema. Next, I present the story of researchers from the Federal University of the São Francisco Valley and the State University of Bahia, founders of the neo-shamanic group Alma, who gather in the Serra dos Morgados to drink jurema wine and sing the simple and beautiful songs "received" (composed) by Juracy Marques and set to music by Edésio César. With Marques, Alexandre Barreto, and Guilherme Medeiros, I learned a bit more about the long and painful struggle of the indigenous peoples of the Northeast against colonial oppression and navigated the deep waters of jurema in a terreiro in Petrolina, retracing the journey I had undertaken months earlier in a neo-shamanic ceremony guided by the catimbozeiro Rômulo Angélico in Natal, in the same Redinha neighborhood where Mário de Andrade underwent a body-closing ritual in 1928, in a Catimbó session.

By this point in my exploration of the Jurema universe, I already had indications that its reign extended beyond the Northeast, although it was nowhere near as ubiquitous or as prominent as the ayahuasca churches born in Northern Brazil. It was, and to some extent still is, a mystery to me why this other religion based on a psychedelic sacrament, so Brazilian and so much more accessible than rituals practiced in the remote Amazon, has not achieved the same penetration in the alternative scene of the urban centers of the Southeast. One possible explanation is that, being so mixed, it diverges from the romantic ideal of Indigenous purity at the heart of the forest—something that ayahuasca religions are not, either. In any case, even if less visible and widespread, Jurema Sagrada was at least present in Belo Horizonte, at the Tenda de Umbanda Caboclo Pena Branca and Casa de Catimbó Mestre Junqueiro, and in the metropolitan area of São Paulo, at Espaço Jurema Mestra in the municipality of Santo André. Despite the closer proximity compared to Alhandra or Baía da Traição, it proved necessary to navigate winding paths to finally attend ceremonies at these two terreiros, respectively a baptism and a Festa das Mestras, with the blessings of Orestes Mineiro and Paulo Alcântara—events that occupy most of the chapter "The Eternal Return of Mysticism."

More idiosyncratic, on the other hand, is the phenomenon of neo-psychodelic churches that consecrate black jurema at the core of their doctrine. Congregations of this type have long proliferated in the United States, as historian J. Christian Greer reports, though not with the institutionalized reach of Santo Daime or União do Vegetal in Brazil and abroad, gathering small groups of devotees around a consciousness-altering sacrament, which may be the psilocybin of "magic" mushrooms or the DMT of ayahuasca—as in the case of the Church of the Eagle and the Condor, which in early 2024 was recognized by American agencies as having the right to commune with the brew, the first non-Christian religion in the USA to be granted such permission. In Brazil, and once again in the Northeast, I found two such emerging religions centered on black jurema, even smaller in scale.

The first is called the Church of the Divine Master on Earth (IDMT, as in the Portuguese acronym), is headquartered in Fortaleza and has a single member: Mark Ian Collins, a philosopher who spent several years on a bureaucratic pilgrimage to legalize a temple that still has no physical location, but is intended to administer DMT extracted from *Mimosa tenuiflora* to people of any faith. I recount the unlikely story of Collins and his follower Jan Clefferson Costa de Freitas, who, together with a group of fifteen friends, founded the Igreja Mirífica Eterna, or the Psychedelic Order of the Divine Tryptamine Molecule, in a suburb of Natal, inspired by the example of the IDMT in Ceará and the scientific-metaphysical speculations of Strassman.

Next, I delve deeper into the attempt to understand the recurring emergence of psychedelic churches and the close association between altered states of consciousness and mysticism, as nurtured in the tradition of perennialism—a way of conceiving religious manifestations that dates back to William James and Aldous Huxley and links them to a universal drive for transcendence, even if, in appearance, they diverge greatly in doctrine and ritual. With Greer's help, I was already beginning to question the true universality of this transcendentalism and the very congruence of psychedelia with mysticism, which seemed so ill-fitted to the practices of Jurema Sagrada I was coming to know and to my own experiences with DMT and other consciousness-altering substances.

After all, what would be the purpose of scientific journalism and this book, if not to provoke thought and prompt a reassessment of worldviews through reflection on important and intriguing facts of nature and culture that shed light on all that surrounds the fascinating Jurema? Such questions gave rise to "Life Lessons and Wisdom from the Ancestors of All Beings," in which I conclude the narrative of this journalistic endeavor by seeking to draw lessons from three years immersed in the realm of Jurema—the power plant, the psychoactive brew, the rituals and gatherings, the Cabocla and her retinue of enchanted beings.

The impact of black jurema on me, however, was not limited to my journey as a reporter. Experiencing firsthand the many practices surrounding Jurema, tracing its roots in Brazilian history, and reflecting deeply on them led to a more open attitude toward the science of Indigenous peoples and their plants, as well as a more critical stance toward a certain unexamined arrogance among biomedical researchers. This impulse to question could not, for the sake of intellectual honesty, exclude an examination of the consequences of all this for my own profession—journalism—and the philosophical questions that the science of Jurema planted in me. This is the purpose of the last chapter, seek truth, act independently, minimize harm which claims for this long account of discoveries in the enchanted science of Jurema the observance of the triad of maxims that should guide the work of every reporter and investigator.

The philosophical exploration that follows is not a digression, but rather a shift in gear, allowing the wheels of the spirit to run more freely along new paths of thought. In the first excursion, I confronted the question that arises for any journalist writing about traditional cultures: how appropriate is it to apply the criteria of science to Indigenous cosmologies in order to define what constitutes reliable knowledge? My longstanding fascination with the writings of the Brazilian anthropologist Eduardo Viveiros de Castro and his generous ideas on Amerindian perspectivism had already shown me that the dichotomy between nature and society makes no sense in this other way of seeing and living in the world, which, in its own way, is also present in the Jurema tradition. Through his influence, I arrived at the mature work of Marshall Sahlins, the spellbinding posthumous book *The New Science of the Enchanted Universe*, in which he prescribes balancing, with grace and confidence, on the tightrope between rigorous research and the sincere acceptance of other epistemologies, without relegating the worldviews "of most of humanity" to the status of belief, magic, primitive animism, or any other subordinate category of colonial anthropology.

The next journey led me to a critical inquiry into the very intertwining of the revived psychedelic science with mystical conceptions—that is, those blind spots of empirical research where it betrays its own assumptions of objectivity and impartiality. It is not new that at least some researchers in the field emphasize the supposedly mystical component of the psychedelic experience, starting with the patriarch of the so-called Psychedelic Renaissance, Roland Griffiths of Johns Hopkins University in the United States. Guided by Greer and Benjamin Breen, I followed the thread that entangles altered states of consciousness with metaphysics and unraveled the skein that links the thought of Huxley to that of Margaret Mead and Gregory Bateson—a journey in which I even encountered Carl Sagan and his visit to a research laboratory in the Caribbean where LSD was administered to dolphins.

Phytolatry—the worship, present in various cultures, that attributes the possession of spirits to trees, of which Jurema Sagrada is a prime example— emerged in the caatinga landscape with a problem that is, in a way, even thornier (no pun intended, given the Tupi etymology of the plant's name, which refers to many thorns): are plants endowed with something that could be compared to thought, agency, or the capacity to perceive the world and respond consistently to what they encounter in order to survive, maybe even some basal form of knowledge?

These are the radical challenges that science and philosophy established themselves in the works of researchers and thinkers such as Stefano Mancuso, Paco Calvo, and Michael Marder, who follow the path first opened by none other than Charles Darwin in his studies of plant behavior and intentionality, in what could be called plant-thinking (*Plant-Thinking* is the title of a thought-provoking book by Marder, subtitled *A Philosophy of Vegetal Life*). With these authors, Western knowledge comes full circle and dares to move toward indigenous cosmogonies that make room for power plants and teacher plants, from which one can learn something about the place of animals and humans in the cosmos.

"The *setting* [the environment in which the psychedelic experience takes place] should be grounded not only in careful intentions but also in a wider sociocultural context that is open to the idea that sacred plants have agency and spirit," recommend Adana Omágua Kambeba, Beatriz Caiuby Labate, and Sidarta Ribeiro.

> Of course, the ontological adoption of Indigenous shamanic cosmologies cannot be 'prescribed', but psychiatry must acknowledge that, by immersing oneself in intricate Indigenous ceremonies and traditions involving sacred plants, one may enhance healing and find a deep sense of belonging and meaning that cannot be disregarded.[1]

Finally, the surprising journey of the last chapter led into the realm of philosophy, the late discipline of thought that, as Friedrich Hegel's saying about the owl of Minerva goes, only takes flight when the shades of night are gathering. What consequences do altered states of consciousness have for the life of the spirit, given their influence on thinkers such as William James, Aldous Huxley, and Ernst Jünger? In closing the book, I echo the call of Peter Sjöstedt-Hughes, from the University of Exeter, for the current Psychedelic Renaissance to mature with the contribution of more rigorous reflection on its premises, aided by philosophy, if only to refine its confused conceptions bundled under the expression "mystical experience," drawing on centuries of systematized metaphysical thought. Sjöstedt-Hughes has even developed a Metaphysical Matrix Questionnaire (MMQ) to assist psychedelic patients and psychotherapists in the laborious task of understanding the notions and insights triggered under the influence of psychoactives, distinguishing, for example, idealism from monism, pantheism from emergentism, and so on.

Along this path, in addition to the teachings of Spinoza on God-Nature received through Sjöstedt-Hughes, I have benefited from the sharp reflections of Nicholas Langlitz and Chris Letheby on the relevance and challenges of distinguishing between methodological naturalism and metaphysical naturalism—a pitfall into which more than one scientist has already stumbled, whether by smuggling mystical notions into their empirical studies or by maintaining a questionable double accounting, taking refuge in a simulated objectivity to better conceal from the public the very metaphysical convictions that encourage them to remain active in a minefield such as psychedelic science, where there have been and will continue to be explosions like the one that, in 2024, blew up the application by the company Lykos to the Food and Drug Administration (FDA), in the United States, to authorize psychotherapy with MDMA for the treatment of post-traumatic stress disorder.

After accompanying me on this journey through a universe as fascinating as it is little known, I invite the reader to judge whether I have managed to rise to its heights.

São Paulo, Brazil   Marcelo Leite, PhD

Note

1. "Psychedelic Science and Indigenous Shamanism: An Urgent Dialogue." *Nature Mental Health*, Oct 26, 2023. p. 815.

Acknowledgments

This book would not exist without the calm dedication of Dráulio de Barros Araújo to psychedelic science and his appreciation for science journalism and communication. When he sought me out in São Paulo in the last week of 2021, he brought as a Christmas gift the seed of DMT in Jurema Sagrada—the plant, the brew, the religion, the science, the cabocla. I owe to him and to Juliana Barreto, his partner, many hours and days of good conversations, good food, warm hospitality, and positive energy. The same goes for the tireless team at the Brain Institute, to whom I extend special thanks, especially to Fernanda Palhano-Fontes, Nicole Galvão-Coelho, Marcelo Falchi, Isabel Wießner, Lucas Maia, and Bruno Lobão. Although not directly related to black jurema, the conversations in Natal with Sidarta Ribeiro and Luiza Mugnol-Ugarte also yielded many ideas, insights, and joys.

All of them, in one way or another, were already present in the making of my previous book, *Psiconautas*, in the inspired company of Bia Labate, Stevens Rehen, and Luís Fernando Tófoli, who for this very reason have also left their mark on the present work. Still within the field of the human and natural sciences, I owe much—almost everything here—to the social scientists Rodrigo Grünewald, Sandro Guimarães de Salles, Luiz Assunção, Estêvão Palitot, Dilaine Sampaio, Guilherme Medeiros, and Miguel Bittencourt, to whom I am grateful for the time and patience invested in long interviews and brief encounters. From afar, through the essential books that quenched my thirst for knowledge, I engaged in dialogue about histories and cosmologies with Eduardo Viveiros de Castro, Marshall Sahlins, Ronaldo

Vainfas, Jeremy Narby, Mário de Andrade, Luís da Câmara Cascudo, René Vandezande, Clarice Novaes da Mota, Clélia Moreira Pinto, Luiz Antonio Simas, and Reginaldo Prandi.

In reflecting on the philosophical and epistemological implications of the traditional and scientific uses of DMT from black jurema, the subject of the final chapters, I turned to the works of researchers of the caliber of Michael Marder, Stefano Mancuso, Paco Calvo, Peter Sjöstedt-Hughes, Chris Letheby, and J. Christian Greer. To them I owe the decisive encouragement to once again savor the delights of that altered state of consciousness called philosophy.

All the information and knowledge accumulated in physical and virtual libraries, however, would be of little or no value without the testimonies gathered among the peoples and communities who consecrate *Mimosa tenuiflora* in Indigenous, rural, and urban areas. To them—the holders of the original science of Jurema—goes my deepest gratitude (in order of appearance in the chapters): Nayanne Alves dos Santos, Raquel Néri de Freitas (Dona Raquel), João José da Silva (Mestre Ciriaco), Severina Paulino de Souza (Mestra Nina), Lucas Paulino de Souza, Eriberto Carvalho Ribeiro (Pai Beto de Xangô), Alexandre L'Omi L'Odó, Joanah Flor, Edézia Maria da Conceição Feitoza (Dona Deza), Afonso Enéas, Elaine Patrícia de Sousa Oliveira (Patrícia Pankararé), Abdon dos Santos (Xixiá Fulni-ô), Rangel Lúcio de Matos (Ytoá Fulni-ô), Isaias Marculino da Silva (Guarapirá), Manuel Pedro dos Santos (Manezinho), Maria das Dores dos Santos (Dorinha), Alessandra Rossi, Paulo de Azevedo (Purna), Alexandre Franca Barreto, Juracy Marques, Rômulo Angélico, Orestes Mineiro, Paulo Alcântara, Margarida Tapeba, Maria Salete Pessoa Guimarães, Mark Ian Collins, and Jan Clefferson Costa de Freitas.

I cannot fail to express my gratitude, above all and beyond my own convictions, to the Mestras and Mestres of Jurema who broke through the Cartesian armor to touch my heart: Zé Pelintra, Zé Bebim, Malunguinho, Cigana, Capitão, and Ritinha.

Many other people contributed to the realization of this book. At *Folha de S.Paulo*, where many of the reports that gave it substance originated, the support of Sérgio Dávila, Vinicius Mota, Roberto Dias, and Marcos Augusto Gonçalves was crucial. At Fósforo publishing house, I once again relied on the steady hand of Rita Mattar and the careful reading of Juliana de Araújo Rodrigues and Bonie Santos, without whom this work would be far less clear and readable. At home, with the affection and understanding of Claudia Kober, my partner of more than four decades, who read all the chapters in their initial versions and gave decisive suggestions to make them more palatable, and of my daughters Ana Kober and Paula Leite (who also read the first manuscript). I dedicate this book to this trio of strong women, in the company of my grandchildren Alice, Tomás, Antônio, and Marina.

Timeline

1580—Santidade de Jaguaripe in the Recôncavo Baiano, a manifestation of religious resistance to colonial domination, already with elements of syncretism between Indigenous rituals and European spiritual traditions.[1]

1640—The German Zacharias Wagener paints *The Calundu dance*, in Pernambuco, considered one of the earliest iconographic records of syncretism between African rituals, Indigenous pajelança, and Catholicism.

1671—French priest Martin de Nantes lives among the Kariri in Paraíba and reports on sorcerers who gave young people a bitter herbal juice to enhance their hunting and fishing skills.

1720—First nominal mention of jurema in a denunciation to the Holy Office.

1741—Letter from the governor of the captaincy of Pernambuco recounts the arrest of Canindé indigenous sorcerers from the village of Boa Vista, with "visions," enemies of the church, and mention of jurema.

1743—Letter from Friar José de Calvatam provides details of the Jurema ritual in Corema villages.

1749—Construction of the Church of Our Lady of the Assumption in Alhandra, followed by a Franciscan friary.

1756—Friar Fidelis de Partana interrogates three Paiacu indigenous people considered sorcerers who used jurema and maracás.

1757—Portuguese Marquis of Pombal creates the Directorate of Indians to oversee them, according to the 1755 law enacted by King José I.

1758—Direct prohibition of Jurema. Indigenous man named Antônio arrested and executed in Mepibu for practicing "adjunto de jurema."

1758—Creation of the village of Alhandra, by order of the Pombaline Directorate.

1762—Creation of the villages of São Miguel da Baía da Traição and Monte-Mor da Preguiça, former Potiguara Indigenous settlements.

1765—Aratagui settlement established as a village under the name Alhandra.

1775—Portuguese King José I elevates settlements to villages under the jurisdiction of the Directorate of Indians.

1779—Physician José dos Santos denounces sorcerers José Pereira, Manuel Lira, and Francisco to the Holy Office for jurema use and "diabolical illusions."

1781—Denunciation against Francisco Pessoa, captain-major of the village of Camaleão, accused of cooking an image of Christ in jurema root water in the company of Indigenous people.

1832—Fulni-ô Indigenous people donate part of their land for the construction of the Church of Our Lady of the Conception, in what is now the city of Águas Belas.

1835—Death of João Batista, last Malunguinho leader of the Catucá quilombo.

1836–38—Jurema sect in Pedra Bonita carries out the alleged sacrifice of 43 people in the Catolé mountains.

1850—Imperial Land Law abolishes settlements, integrates them into emerging towns, and opens the way for land leases.

1865—Writer José de Alencar mentions the jurema wine in the novel *Iracema*.

1865—Antonio Gonçalves da Justa Araújo demarcates plots for Indigenous families in Alhandra.

1908—Zélio Fernandino de Morais incorporates Caboclo das Sete Encruzilhadas during a spiritualist session in Rio de Janeiro, marking the beginning of Kardecist Umbanda.

1910—Maria Eugênia (Maria do Acais 2) returns from Recife to Alhandra after inheriting the estate of Maria Gonçalves de Barros (Maria do Acais 1), sister of Ignácio Gonçalves de Barros, shaman and last "regent of the Indians."

1920—Indian Protection Service (SPI) begins recognition of Indigenous lands in the Northeast of Brazil

1927—Ascenso Ferreira publishes the poetry book *Catimbó*, which draws the attention of folklorist Mário de Andrade.

1928—Mário de Andrade has his body "closed" by catimbozeiros in Natal.

1931—German-Canadian chemist Richard Manske synthesizes the compound N,N -dimethyltryptamine (DMT).

1932—Maria do Acais 2 builds a chapel for Saint John the Baptist.

1937—Death of Maria do Acais 2.

1938—Gonçalves Fernandes publishes *O Folclore Mágico do Nordeste*, with the chapter "As mesas de Catimbó, ritual mágico," in which he recounts the biography of Maria do Acais.

1938—Folklore Research Mission, organized by Mário de Andrade, records several Catimbó chants in the Northeast.

1939—First Umbanda Federation in Brazil.

1941—First Congress of Spiritism and Umbanda.

1945—Roger Bastide publishes *Imagens do Nordeste Místico em Preto e Branco*, in which he presents Catimbó as of Indigenous origin.

1946—Oswaldo Gonçalves de Lima publishes the article "Observações sobre o 'vinho da Jurema' utilizado pelos índios Pancarú de Tacaratú (Pernambuco)" and reports the isolation of the psychoactive substance he calls nigerine (DMT).

1951—Luís da Câmara Cascudo publishes *Meleagro*, about Catimbó.

1956—Hungarian chemist and psychiatrist Stephen Szara injects dimethyl-tryptamine into his own body and confirms the psychedelic effect of DMT.

1957—First Assembly of God evangelical temple in Alhandra.

1959—Death of Flósculo, son of Maria do Acais.

1966—Law no. 3,443 of Paraíba guarantees religious freedom and creates the Federation of African Cults.

1971—U.S. President Richard Nixon declares the War on Drugs, which will lead to the prohibition of psychedelic substances in almost the entire world.

1975—René Vandezande defends his master's *Catimbó. Pesquisa Exploratória sobre a Forma Nordestina de Religião Mediúnica*.

1985—MDMA (ecstasy) is added to the list of prohibited substances in the USA

1993—American pharmacologist Jonathan Ott publishes *Pharmacotheon*, a compendium on psychedelics, which he calls entheogens, with special emphasis on DMT.

2000—Richard Strassman releases the book *DMT: The Spirit Molecule.*

2006—First Kipupa Malunguinho festival in Pernambuco, organized by Alexandre L'Omi L'Odó.

2006—Luiz Assunção publishes the book *O Reino dos Mestres. A tradição da jurema na umbanda nordestina.*

2006—Roland Griffiths, from Johns Hopkins University, publishes the pioneering article "Psilocybin can occasion mystical-type experiences with substantial and sustained personal meaning and spiritual significance."

2007—The process to declare Acais a protected heritage site begins at the Institute of Historical and Artistic Heritage of the State of Paraíba.

2007—Malunguinho Law (Municipal Law no. 13,298, Recife) establishes the Municipal Week of Experience and Practice of Afro-Indigenous Pernambucan Culture.

2008—Rodrigo Grünewald publishes the chapter "Jurema e Novas Religiosidades Metropolitanas" in the book *Índios do Nordeste: Etnia, Política e História.*

2009—Peace March, in defense of a "city" (sacred tree) of Jurema, takes place on June 20 in Alhandra.

2009—Acais is declared a protected heritage site on September 30, but the house had already been demolished by order of the owner.

2009—Victory March in Alhandra, on November 15, celebrates the heritage listing of Acais, although only the Chapel of Saint John the Baptist survived.

2010—Sandro Guimarães de Salles publishes the book *À Sombra da Jurema Encantada. Mestres juremeiros na Umbanda de Alhandra.*

2012—Guilherme Medeiros defends at the University of Clermont-Ferrand his doctoral thesis *L'Usage Rituel de la Jurema chez les Amérindiens du Brésil: Répression et Survie des Coutumes Indigènes à l'Époque de la Conquête Spirituelle Européenne (XVIeme-XVIIeme Siècles).*

2012—Neuroscientist Dráulio de Araújo publishes, with collaborators from THE UNIVERSITY OF SÃO PAULO in Ribeirão Preto, the article. "Seeing with the eyes shut: Neural basis of enhanced imagery following ayahuasca ingestion."

2017—Alexandre L'Omi L'Odó defends his master's dissertation *Juremologia: Uma Busca Etnográfica para Sistematização de Princípios da Cosmovisão da Jurema Sagrada.*

2018—Araújo publishes with colleagues from UFRN the pioneering article "Antidepressant Effects of the Psychedelic Ayahuasca in Treatment-Resistant Depression: A Randomized Placebo-Controlled Trial," on the therapeutic effect of DMT.

2021—Araújo Group at the Brain Institute launches the Dunas Project to investigate inhalation of the psychedelic DMT from black jurema for depression.

2024—Araújo group publishes the article "The Antidepressant Effects of Vaporized N,N -dimethyltryptamine: an open-label trial in treatment-resistant depression," presenting clinical trial results.

2024—The U.S. Food and Drug Administration rejects the application for the use of MDMA to treat post-traumatic stress disorder, delaying the legalization of psychedelic therapies in the USA.

Note

1. This chronology, not being the work of a historian, does not claim to be exhaustive, but merely to illustrate the parallel occurrence of religious, social, cultural, and scientific events related to Jurema and DMT.

Contents

The Goddess Jurema and the Devil of Science Against the Dragon of Anxiety

The scene is unusual: on a morning in 2022, a neuroscientist and a former senator venture into the Brazilian northeastern backlands to uproot trees. In 45 min, with the help of a tractor, rope, hoe, and chainsaw, three specimens of black jurema (*Mimosa tenuiflora*) are extracted with their roots intact, as planned.[1] The roots contain the highest concentration of N,N-dimethyltryptamine (DMT), the reason for the agro-scientific expedition. This consciousness-altering substance is among the most promising new drugs to help patients whom psychiatry today cannot always treat, such as those suffering from post-traumatic stress disorder (PTSD) and depression resistant to conventional treatments—a turning point in mental health since the turn of the century, known as the Psychedelic Renaissance, led by MDMA (ecstasy)[2] and the psilocybin found in "magic" mushrooms.

The owner of the Logradouro farm in Quixadá, state of Ceará, is Flávio Torres de Araújo, 77 years old at the time of the visit, a physicist and founder of the Democratic Labor Party (PDT) in Ceará. As the alternate for Senator Patricia Saboya, he served as a member of parliament for four months in 2009. He also owns a BMW 1200 motorcycle, on which he would soon depart for a trip to Peru. Like his father, Dráulio Barros de Araújo is a physicist and holds a doctorate in physics applied to medicine and biology from the University of São Paulo (USP). At fifty, he has spent fifteen years researching psychoactive substances such as the DMT found in ayahuasca. Studies by his team on the antidepressant effects of the brew have helped place Brazil third in the ranking of most impactful articles in the psychedelic science renaissance,[3] according to a survey published in 2021 by David Wyndham Lawrence.[4]

M. Leite, *The Psychedelic Science of the Jurema Tree*, Copernicus Books, https://doi.org/10.1007/978-3-032-22705-8_1

It had rained all night on May 21. The waterlogged soil offered little resistance to the removal of the black jurema roots, the dominant tree in that stretch of caatinga. Father and son worked alongside the manager, José Edson Pereira da Silva, 49, who drove the Massey Ferguson tractor. The reddish taproot, sections of the darkened trunk, compound leaves with several leaflets, and a few white flowers were separated for transport to Natal (state of Rio Grande do Norte), about five hundred kilometers away. There, they would be processed at the Brain Institute of the Federal University of Rio Grande do Norte (ICe-UFRN). The lower parts of each tree's trunk, still with secondary roots, were returned to the soil. The idea is for them to sprout again, giving rise to new plants and restarting the life cycle in the caatinga, which turns green when the rains arrive.

After the collection, the next stop was at the ranch near the reservoir at the farm headquarters, at the foot of the enormous Pedra da Pendência. This porphyritic granite block is part of the impressive regional set of Quixadá monoliths, *inselbergs* (island mountains) that dot the landscape. The lakeside appetizer menu featured curimatã roe seasoned with tomato, bell pepper, and herbs. To drink, cachaça from a French oak barrel and beer. The neuroscientist emerged from the water, where small fish nibbled at the bathers' feet, and, passing by his father, kissed him on the forehead. He asked him to tell another story, like the one about the trip when he took his eleven-year-old son fishing on the Araguaia River.

Higher up, the 1932 house is rustic, with no ceiling lining. Flávio Torres, as the former senator is better known, bought the property in 1983. The family traveled there frequently from Fortaleza. "Much of my personality was shaped here on this farm," his son recounts. Heir inheriting his father's adventurous spirit, he has already practiced deep-sea diving and skydiving; today, he is dedicated to surfing. Every month, around the 20th, Araújo the son travels the thousand-kilometer round trip between Natal and Quixadá. He aims to characterize the plant *Mimosa tenuiflora* in each season of the year, particularly the DMT content in its various parts. He is searching for clues about the function of the molecule in the plant's physiology.

Black jurema is an abundant and inexpensive source of the psychedelic, which is extracted in the researcher's laboratory at the ICe. Its roots have been used for centuries in Indigenous and Afro-Brazilian rituals. The DMT molecule became the subject of experiments at the university, initiated in June 2021, to verify and quantify its antidepressant effect when administered by inhalation. Healthy volunteers received doses, and the results—which showed that the inhaled formulation is safe and produces the intended psychedelic effect—served as the basis for designing the actual experiment with patients suffering from treatment-resistant depression, recruited at the Onofre Lopes University Hospital (HUOL) of the UFRN.

"Why does DMT occur so widespread in living beings?" asks Dráulio, seated on the long veranda of the Logradouro farm. His hypothesis, in the case of animals, is that dimethyltryptamine is the engine behind the images that arise in dreams, or the closed-eye visions and "mirações" described by ayahuasca users. The expression became the title of one of his pioneering scientific articles on the psychedelic, "Seeing with the Eyes Shut," published in 2012.[5] Functional magnetic resonance imaging records have revealed that the visions triggered by ayahuasca stem from the activation of an extensive neural network involved in vision, memory, and intention. "Many effects are very similar to what happens when a person is dreaming. We see our own thoughts, we gain access to our own emotions," says the neuroscientist, who has himself experienced ayahuasca (not always peacefully).

Even more mysterious is the widespread occurrence of DMT in plants. Dráulio speculates that the compound may have a more fundamental biological function, such as preparing organisms for environmental stress, for example, the long droughts of the caatinga. His practice of collecting black jurema samples every month is related to this idea. He wants to establish how the dimethyltryptamine content varies in each part of the tree during the northeastern summer (dry season) and winter (rainy season), in search of clues about the molecule's function.

A broader characteristic under investigation by the UFRN research group is the anti-inflammatory effect that DMT shares with other psychedelics. Since increased levels of inflammation are found in depressed patients, the antidepressant benefit of the molecule may also be linked to its ability to reduce brain inflammation, and not only to the access to remote psychic content it enables during the psychedelic experience. Another factor fueling Dráulio's scientific imagination comes from studies showing the ability of psychedelics, including DMT, to activate metabolic pathways associated with the formation of new neural connections. This is known as neuroplasticity. By opening new pathways for the exchange of impulses between neurons, DMT could foster the emergence of thoughts capable of breaking the vicious cycles of negative ideas—the rumination that torments those with severe depression. Neuroplasticity would thus be another process contributing to the antidepressant effect.

A fan of science fiction films such as *Dune* and following the suggestion of psychiatrist Marcelo Falchi, Dráulio Araújo named the initiative Project Dunas (also a reference to the typical sand dunes of the coast in Rio Grande do Norte). But the researcher also likes to refer to it as "DMT from A to

Z." One of the enigmas that the systematic study of *Mimosa tenuiflora* may unravel is the effect of the so-called "jurema wine," consumed ceremonially by Indigenous groups in the Northeast. At least in the recipes used today, the brew seems to lack a decisive element for the psychedelic effect to occur: a compound capable of preventing the degradation of DMT during digestion, without which the psychoactive does not reach the brain. In ayahuasca, for example, this inhibitor is provided by the mariri vine, or jagube. Could jurema-preta itself provide these inhibitors? So far, it is speculated that such blockers may be present in other plants that, in certain preparation recipes, are added to the ceremonial drink, such as wild varieties of cashew and passion fruit—fruits not used everywhere the wine is made. It may be that this mystery has no biochemical solution. However, it cannot be ruled out that access to the enchanted realms of the Sacred Jurema is opened by the rituals themselves, without direct psychedelic influence.

Black jurema-preta is just one of the 38 species of the genus *Mimosa* found in the caatinga (out of 350 in Brazil, among 540 worldwide). Some also contain DMT, but *Mimosa tenuiflora* has become the preferred species for rituals. This may be due to its high DMT content or its ubiquity in the northeastern backlands. The hardiness of jurema is even reflected in its name, which means "many thorns" in the Indigenous language Tupi. Even in a semi-arid environment, it can reach up to 5.5 m in height and thirty centimeters in trunk diameter.[6] Its dominance in the caatinga landscape is attributed to its unusual tolerance to different soil conditions and water deficits. During drought, it loses all its leaves, which return green with the first rains. White flowers usually appear between November and December. The high tannin content, which gives the drink made from jurema its bitterness, does not prevent cattle and goats from feeding on its shoots in the rainy season and on its leaves and pods during the dry season. Its wood is more dense than eucalyptus, making it the preferred choice among locals for fence posts and charcoal production.

As a legume, it harbors nitrogen-fixing bacteria in its roots through symbiosis, enriching the nutrient-poor soils of the caatinga with this essential element. It is a suitable tree for reforestation, as it grows rapidly—4.5 m in five years—and 75% of seedlings survive during this period. Nevertheless, all this resilience may not be enough to withstand the increasing human presence in the backlands. Nearly half (46%) of the caatinga biome has already been deforested,[7] 10.5% of it between 1985 and 2021 alone. The surface area of water—rivers and reservoirs—in the biome shrank by 16.8% in the same period, putting several areas at risk of desertification.[8]

Despite its abundance, black jurema is not immune to this wave of devastation. According to a genetic study by Sendi Reis Arruda of the State University of Southwest Bahia (UESB), fragmentation of the caatinga is already reducing gene flow between separated populations of *Mimosa tenuiflora*.[9] Without proper pollen and seed dispersal, the trees reproduce only with nearby conspecifics, confined to the same area. This reduces the genetic diversity available to make the plant more robust in the face of varying environmental conditions. Over time, this loss of diversity could threaten the survival of the species.

Observing Dráulio and Flávio harvesting just three jurema-preta trees from the vast juremal on the Logradouro farm in Quixadá, one might think it makes little difference to the population of this tree in the northeastern semi-arid region. After all, at a rate of three specimens per month to obtain a few hundred milligrams of DMT, that would be only 36 trees in a year. However, father and son take care to return the stumps of the three trees, along with their secondary roots, to the soil so they can sprout again and help restore the vigor of the caatinga. In this act, they also renew the bond between them and the hope that studies with DMT will help alleviate the suffering of millions with depression.

Nigerine, the Indigenous Secret in the Sacred Wine of the Pankararu

Brazilian science, especially in the Northeast, has a long history with the DMT molecule. The natural alkaloid was first isolated and described by a chemist from Pernambuco, Oswaldo Gonçalves de Lima (1908–1989), who extracted it from jurema-preta in the 1940s. It was the dark color of the caatinga tree's trunk that inspired him to name it "nigerine." As the first director of the School of Chemistry, later incorporated into the Federal University of Pernambuco (UFPE), Gonçalves de Lima founded, in 1952, the Institute of Antibiotics at the University of Recife, also later absorbed by the same university. He published 228 scientific articles, 29 of them in international journals.[10] One of these articles established his name in the psychedelic scientific literature: "Observações sobre o 'vinho da Jurema' utilizado pelos índios Pancarú de Tacaratú (Pernambuco)."[11]

Gonçalves de Lima had many interests, ranging from politics—he was imprisoned for two months in 1935 after the Intentona Comunista (Communist Uprising)—to German literature, as evidenced by a 1965 inaugural lecture titled "Goethe e a Química."[12] He was also a defender of the

Indigenous peoples of the Americas and an admirer of Indigenous rights advocates Marshal Cândido Mariano da Silva Rondon and anthropologist Darcy Ribeiro. In October 1942, the chemist visited a village of the ethnic group now known as the Pankararu in Jatobá, in the backlands of Pernambuco. He was accompanied by students and technicians for geological studies in the São Francisco River valley.

In his article, Gonçalves de Lima recounts his frustration at not having witnessed the ajucá ceremony, the sacred wine made there from black jurema. He only observed the preparation of the beverage by the juremeiro Serafim Joaquim dos Santos. Shavings of the macerated root are squeezed in cold water, which turns red and foamy. After the foam is removed, the clay vessel receives pipe smoke blown over it in the shape of a cross. Having not witnessed the trance induced by the wine during the rituals, Gonçalves de Lima quotes the ethnographer Carlos Estevão de Oliveira: "At that moment, they gave the impression that the leaden blade of pseudo-civilization we have spread over them, though four centuries thick, is far too light to smother their beliefs." The chemist notes the Indigenous influence on the Catimbó cults in Pernambuco and the Candomblé de Caboclo in Bahia. The major contribution was jurema, the epicenter of the "rather limited phytolatry of the Indians of the Northeast," which "only became a sacred tree when it was identified as a delightful means of transport." (English translations by the author).

With the samples obtained, Gonçalves de Lima applied various chemical methods to extract nigerine, the transporting alkaloid. This was the first record of DMT in natural organisms, but it later became clear that the same substance had been synthesized in 1931 by the Canadian chemist Richard Manske.[13] The confirmation that N,N-dimethyltryptamine was responsible for the psychedelic effect came only in 1956, when the Hungarian chemist and psychiatrist Stephen Szara[14] injected DMT into his own muscle and, well… tripped. Gonçalves de Lima, on the other hand, reports that a member of his team ingested 40 mg of nigerine and experienced only increased pulse, heightened auditory perception, and respiratory symptoms (mild dyspnea), without any psychedelic effect, certainly due to the absence of digestive enzyme inhibitors. All these phenomena disappeared within 45 min, he recorded.

In 1965, decades after nigerine was isolated, an article in the journal *The Alabama Journal of Medical Science*[15] reported a surprising fact: a form of DMT is present in the healthy human brain, even without the ingestion of psychoactive substances. In other words, dimethyltryptamine is produced locally in the very organ upon which it exerts psychedelic effects when introduced from outside. This discovery would provide a strong argument in favor of the idea that DMT, being endogenous, is likely to be a safe drug, should its therapeutic utility be proven. Of course, it would be necessary to test the range of doses that could be used safely. With the popularity gained by ayahuasca among hippies, with works such as *The Yagé Letters* (another name for the Amazonian brew), by William S. Burroughs and Allen Ginsberg, already in 1966, just three years after the book's publication, the first restrictions on its use in research appeared.[16]

DMT is found not only in black jurema, in the chacruna shrub used in ayahuasca, and in the human brain, but also in other animals, plants, and even fungi. A comprehensive overview of its ubiquity can be found in the book *TiHKAL* by Ann and Alexander "Sasha" Shulgin.[17] The couple spent several years synthesizing psychedelics in a home laboratory in California, which they tested in self-experiments with friends. "DMT is, most simply, almost everywhere you choose to look. It is in this flower here, in that tree over there, and in yonder animal." The long section on DMT in the book is first introduced by pointing to a close relative, 5,6-dibromo-DMT, found in the marine sponge *Smenospongia ehina* and in the tunicate *Eudistoma fragum*. N,N-dimethyltryptamine itself appears in a type of coral from the Bay of Naples, *Paramuricea chamaeleon*. The list continues with several species of fungi across seven families. Next come the toads, with 5-hydroxy-DMT (bufotenine) and 5-MeO-DMT.

Moving on to the plant kingdom, Shulgin begins by listing grasses of the genus *Phalaris*, such as *P. tuberosa*, which causes sheep that feed on it to stagger. Another genus of grass toxic to animals is *Lolium*, in addition to various species of bamboo and reeds. Among the legumes, many species from the genera *Acacia*, *Anadenanthera*, and *Mimosa*. From the angico tree *Anadenanthera peregrina* and its relative *A. colubrina*, for example, psychoactive snuffs are extracted in South America, known as paricá, yopo, vilca, huilca, and cebil. There are also trees of the genus *Virola*, whose resin is likewise used to produce snuffs. Finally, and most importantly, in the large psychoactive family of coffee relatives, the ayahuasca plant chacruna, *Psychotria viridis*, is the only one to contain DMT.

The presence of DMT in various plants is also noted in a classic work on psychedelics, *Plants of the Gods*. In a table of "ayahuasca analogues," 21 species from five families are listed: Gramineae, Leguminosae (with *Acacia simplicifolia* and *Mimosa tenuiflora* leading in DMT concentrations, at 0.81% and 0.57–1%, respectively), Malpighiaceae, Myristicaceae, Rubiaceae, and Rutaceae. The authors even provide a recipe for "juremahuasca" or "mimosahuasca": three grams of Syrian rue seeds (*Peganum harmala*), nine grams of black jurema root bark, and the juice of one lemon, recommending that the Syrian rue tea be taken fifteen minutes before the jurema and lemon preparation, so that the first drink inhibits the degradation of the psychoactive DMT in the digestive system.[18]

Pedro Luz also included black jurema in his compendium of 44 psychoactive plants, *Carta psiconáutica*. He describes the plant as a shrub with strong, straight thorns, thick at the base, measuring 5 to 6 mm in length.[19] Luz summarizes the importance of jurema and its wine in the indigenous cultures of the Northeast and reproduces an account of visions caused by consuming tea prepared from the plant and Syrian rue seeds.

A Journey to the Dark and Solitary Depths of the Mind

It is 7:25 a.m. upon arrival at the hospital HUOL, in Natal. The experimenters for the study in which I will be a subject, Fernanda Palhano-Fontes, Marcelo Falchi, Sophie Laborde, Nicole Galvão-Coelho, Isabel Wießner, and Aline Assunção, are already in position. The small room in the hospital basement at UFRN has been decorated to provide comfort for people like me, who are volunteers in this pilot phase of the DMT study. The beige armchair reserved for the human subject is reclining and comfortable. Electroencephalography equipment (EEG), Volcano vaporizer, headphones, and nursing supplies: everything is ready.

They then explain what will happen, recalling previous agreements made during the screening session with Falchi and the preparation session with Laborde. They may, for example, touch my arm or hold my hand, if necessary. They describe the duration and sequence of the experiment: multiple blood and saliva collections, two doses of DMT, one EEG before and another after each peak in the two psychedelic sessions, completion of questionnaires and psychometric scales, and two rapid integration sessions with the psychologist, during which the patient discusses their experiences under the influence of the substance and the meanings or feelings they attribute to them.

The small orchestra is conducted by Dráulio Araújo. He enters the room, checks that everything is in order, and gives the green light. This is the fourth dress rehearsal of the preliminary phase of a clinical trial investigating the antidepressant effect of inhaled DMT. The experiment was set to begin in earnest the following month, June, with the first healthy volunteers (without depression) but with prior experience using psychedelics.

According to the World Health Organization (WHO), about 300 million people worldwide live with depressive disorder, 5% of the adult population.[20] Considering that at least one third of those with depression find no relief with available antidepressants, alternative treatments are sorely needed. The new study continues the research by ICe-UFRN that led, in 2018, to the publication of the world's first placebo-controlled clinical trial in which a psychedelic substance was tested for depression. On that occasion, ayahuasca was used, the religious sacrament of the Santo Daime, Barquinha, and União do Vegetal (UDV) churches, studied mainly at UFRN and the School of Medicine at the Ribeirão Preto campus of the University of São Paulo (USP). Twenty-nine volunteers with treatment-resistant depression participated, fourteen of whom took the brew and fifteen received an active placebo (bitter-tasting and capable of causing gastrointestinal discomfort, to mimic ayahuasca). One week later, after completing standardized questionnaires to assess the severity of depressive symptoms, nine of the fourteen in the ayahuasca group still had lower scores, meaning they were significantly less depressed; in the other group, only four out of fifteen showed improvement.[21] After several attempts with different journals, the corresponding article was eventually published in *Psychological Medicine*.[22]

After that pioneering study, Dráulio spent two sabbatical years at the University of California, Santa Barbara, in the United States. He returned with the project of testing the potential of DMT, isolating the psychoactive compound in ayahuasca believed to be responsible for its antidepressant effect. He was convinced of the need to shorten the psychedelic session for therapeutic purposes. The "force" of the brew, as followers of the Daime religions say, can last three to four hours. Such a long journey would be difficult to accommodate in a clinical setting, as it would require the presence of trained therapists throughout. This would increase the cost of the procedure, if approved, and limit the number of patients who could be treated.

Other psychedelics under investigation for psychiatric disorders present similar challenges. The effect of MDMA for PTSD, for example, can last six hours. This is roughly the same duration of a session with psilocybin, the psychoactive compound in "magic" mushrooms, which is also advancing in clinical trials for depression. Today, there is less research on LSD, not only because of the stigma acquired during the War on Drugs since the 1970s, but also because a lysergic journey can last eight hours or more. If ayahuasca were to be used medically, it would present an additional problem: its preparation varies greatly from place to place, making standardization and dosage control difficult.

Hence the preference of some research groups, such as Dráulio's, for using pure DMT. In the case of ICe UFRN, the compound has been extracted from black jurema, a plant abundant in the caatinga. This northeastern plant has become the primary ingredient in juremahuasca, an ayahuasca analogue widely used by urban neo-shamans in Brazil and Europe. In the Netherlands, for example, juremahuasca was tested in a study at Maastricht University on its antidepressant effect. Published in the journal *Psychopharmacology*,[23] the article found that the benefit persisted for up to one year in twelve out of seventeen participants in neo-shamanic ceremonies seeking help for moderate to severe depression.[24]

When inhaled, dimethyltryptamine produces a short acute effect, lasting ten to fifteen minutes. Absorbed into the bloodstream through the lungs, it reaches the brain quickly, thus bypassing the digestive system, where it would otherwise be inactivated by an enzyme. In its basic form, DMT is insoluble in water and suitable for sublimation—that is, it can transition directly from a solid to a gaseous state, making it possible to smoke in pipes,[25] either mixed with herbs or not, in which case it is known in non-academic circles as *changa*.

Biomind, a company headquartered in the United Kingdom and chaired by Uruguayan entrepreneur Alejandro Antalich, entered into a brief agreement with UFRN to support the clinical trial conducted by the ICe UFRN teams, as well as all research involving extraction and synthesis of DMT and animal testing. The partnership provided funding for the university and the institute as a whole, in addition to resources for Dráulio's laboratory. In Project Dunas, the agreement with Biomind enabled the assembly of a team of twenty people, including psychiatrists, psychologists, chemists, nurses, animal experimenters, and physiologists. These funds were used to set up the laboratory for processing black jurema and the rooms where experiments are conducted. However, in December 2022, the partnership was dissolved.

Project Dunas yielded its first academic result on December 22, 2023, with an article published electronically in the journal *European Neuropsychopharmacology*[26] in which the team reports, based on the experience of 27 healthy volunteers (without depression), that inhaled pure DMT was safe and produced a psychedelic effect proportional to all tested doses. The "trip" induced by inhalation is immediate (beginning within seconds) and brief, making it much more promising for outpatient treatment.

"Our study is pioneering in investigating the effects of DMT administered by inhalation, marking a significant advance in psychedelic research," notes psychiatrist Marcelo Falchi, first author of the study.[27] "We chose a less invasive and more accessible approach, opening new avenues for the therapeutic use of psychedelics," he said at the time of publication. No one experienced serious adverse effects. Only a few mild effects were reported: headache, palpitations, chills, sweating, nausea, etc.—all transient. On fourteen occasions, volunteers also laughed, as recorded in the meticulous Table 2 of the article. "It is very clear to us that DMT administered by inhalation has an effect on mood, and it appears to be positive, with measured items such as affect, arousal, comfort, and satisfaction."

Indeed, as reported by the newspaper *Folha de S.Paulo*,[28] two weeks after this article was published, the ICe-UFRN team released the preliminary results of the evaluation of the first six patients with treatment-resistant depression who underwent experimental treatment with inhaled DMT. The article brought good news: the antidepressant effect was immediate and, after one week, four of the six volunteers were in remission.

The authors compared these results with two other similar studies. One tested DMT for depression in seven participants,[29] but administered it intravenously, with the psychedelic effect lasting up to thirty minutes (when inhaled, the effect lasts ten to fifteen minutes). Another difference: the competing study did not include psychotherapeutic support, as was provided in the UFRN group. The antidepressant benefit of the injection, assessed using standardized scales, was much lower than that of inhalation in the ICe-UFRN group. The second comparison involved a trial using inhalation with the same vaporizer device, Volcano, involving sixteen depressed patients, but with a related substance, 5-MeO-DMT, originally extracted from the venom of the Colorado River toad (*Incilius alvarius*). In this case, the benefit obtained was similar to that of the Brazilian study. Incidentally, 5-MeO-DMT administered nasally is the flagship product of the British company Beckley PsyTech, which originated from the Beckley Foundation, founded by drug decriminalization activist Amanda Feilding. The company, chaired by her son, Cosmo Feilding-Mellen, is developing the BPL-003 formulation of the drug to treat depression and alcohol abuse and, in early 2024, received a $50 million investment from the holding company atai Life Sciences, owned by entrepreneur Christian Angermayer, a proponent of patents for psychedelics. There is no way to draw major conclusions from the three trials, given the small number of participants. However, the experiments suggest that parenteral DMT—that is, not oral, but rather inhaled or injected—is safe and has the potential to treat depression at a lower cost than multi-hour sessions with other psychedelics. Combining the treatment with psychotherapy also appears to be more effective. In fact, on the same January 4, another study measured and confirmed the importance of a strong collaborative relationship between psychotherapist and patient in MDMA-assisted therapy for PTSD. Paradoxically, this association of the compound with psychotherapy ended up constituting one of the main obstacles that led the FDA to reject the psychedelic as a new treatment for PTSD in August 2024.

Placing the white EEG cap, with 32 electrodes, takes some time. Of medium size, it does not fit my head very well. One electrode on the right side is slightly displaced and does not transmit a signal. Another dab of gel reestablishes the conductive bridge between the metal and the scalp, resolving the issue. The intravenous access in the right arm is also challenging. Assunção, the nurse, is unable to draw blood at five and ten minutes, meaning two of the eleven collections fail. She attributes the difficulty to clots forming in the very fine plastic catheter inserted into the blood vessel. Once or twice, blood leaks, and she cleans my arm with alcohol. None of this bothers me, and the information seems to reassure her, given the tension of the tight collection schedule and the risk of hemolysis (when red blood cells rupture under pressure, hindering subsequent centrifugation to separate them from the serum for clinical analysis).

Falchi displays the metal mesh with thirty milligrams of DMT that will go into the Volcano vaporizer. The device, originally developed for medicinal applications of cannabidiol (a medicine derived from cannabis), transforms the DMT into gas and transfers it to a plastic balloon with a mouthpiece that the patient uses to inhale it. After practicing with the balloon three times without the substance, the time comes for the actual inhalation—a lower dose to familiarize the patient with the substance and the apparatus. It is not easy to empty the two-liter reservoir balloon, because DMT irritates the airways, provoking a cough reflex. Successive swallowing reflexes help retain breath for ten seconds after emptying the crinkling plastic balloon, which the psychiatrist squeezes to help direct the gas into the volunteer's lungs. Once the gas is retained in the lungs, the beige armchair is reclined for takeoff. The visual effect is similar to that of changa smoked on Algodões beach (state of Bahia) two months earlier, during the neo-shamanic Equinox festival. Coldness in the arms and the impression that everything is slipping away, with a fainting sensation seeming imminent. An immense lightness, as if floating in space. The onset is dizzying and everything becomes instantly colorful. There is great difficulty in retaining and describing the images: they seem two-dimensional, as if projected onto the screen of closed eyelids, somewhat fractal, but neither geometric nor kaleidoscopic. They are more organic, with curved boundaries between colors, no straight lines or angles. The forms repeat, predominantly in yellow, brown, orange, and red, with little blue, green, or purple. Beautiful, but less dazzling than the images with changa, which on the Bahia beach resembled arabesques in an Istanbul mosque.

Even with the altered perception of time, it is clear that the journey lasts only a few minutes during the visual phase. Someone touches my arm to let me know they are about to record the EEG and ask me to alternate between eyes open and eyes closed. The first recording, five minutes with headphones playing music by Raphael Egel, Wießner's husband, is uneventful, as is the sequence of opening and closing my eyelids. Everything seems amusing, several moments filled with good humor. Many smiles and pleasure. A pleasant experience with those researchers, though not exactly in connection with them, more inwardly focused. Another five minutes with eyes closed, now without music, and it becomes difficult not to fall asleep. Images of an unknown boy appear, fleeting like those seen when slipping into sleep.

After this first dose, I am surprised when the physician, Falchi, says that forty minutes have already passed. He asks if he can proceed to the integration session with psychologist Sophie Laborde and the psychometric scales. Everything sounds amusing, but my reasoning is impaired. I find it somewhat difficult to understand and mark the vertical lines with a red pen on the scale assessing the intensity and quality (pleasant/unpleasant) of the experience.

The second and highest dose of the pilot experiment I participated in at the hospital is the full dose, whose safety and efficacy are being tested—one hundred milligrams in the vaporizer. The onset is somewhat similar and, at the same time, completely different from the first. Someone has already described the experience as launching in a rocket, but clinging to the outside of the vehicle. To begin with, there is intense heat, not cold. Despite the identical volume of gas in the balloon, emptying it proves more difficult. There is intense irritation in the throat and lungs, almost unbearable, forcing me to inhale through my nose without releasing the mouthpiece, swallowing hard to avoid coughing. The ten-second count seems endless, and halfway through, a thunderous vertical ascent begins. The effort required to breathe is much greater, as is the anxiety. Repeatedly opening my eyes is an attempt to dispel the disturbing sense of helplessness. My heart races and systolic blood pressure rises to nearly 170 (with the first dose, it had reached 145).

I need to ask someone to hold my hand while I stroke the fabric on the left armrest of the chair. There are marked differences in the visual effects when comparing the first DMT dose with the second. Everything appears exotically three-dimensional, or perhaps multidimensional, because the transparencies and navigation through the colorful space bear no resemblance to projections on a screen, as if viewed with 3D glasses in a cinema. My disembodied head moves through halls and corridors of palaces, as if it were a drone. The partitions of the spaces traversed display figures reminiscent of alien symbols or scripts vaguely resembling Central American Indigenous writing. The whole setting evokes a spaceship or an environment from another planet, and it would not be surprising if an ET appeared there before me, given the overwhelming sense of imminence.

Once the images dissipate and introspection intensifies, the feeling is no longer one of amusement or delighted astonishment, as it was a few hours earlier, but of heaviness. There is no lightness or floating. The body tenses, not exactly rigid, but contracted. Pressure and mild pain in the head. Stiff neck, as well as jaw. Some involuntary contractions, tremor in the right arm, subtle whole-body spasms. Nothing worrisome, however. The bodily sensations are accompanied by a marked drop in mood. A kind of sadness, not exactly painful; more melancholy than sadness. It is as if there is a disappointed reminder that being alive means being apart from others—ultimately, alone. The abandonment of being an individual, separate, and autonomous.

In the integration conversation that follows, Laborde asks if the feeling is of returning to childhood. In a way, yes, in what is painful and disconcerting. The main insight, as the psychologist hears, comes with the intuition that successive doses trigger contact with two different layers of the psyche. In the first dose, the motivated and determined everyday self is at play, always trying to move forward, look up, make jokes, show affection, seek pleasure, fun, humor, well-being, and productivity. That part that manages to find joy in life, despite everything, despite President Jair Bolsonaro, the pandemic, the previously unsuspected inhumanity in so many Brazilians. In the second dose, there is a descent into a basement of the mind, where a harder, more basic, primitive core resides. Not something dark, desperate, or distressing, but less bright, grounded, immobile like a monolith from Quixadá. It is difficult to find words for such raw emotions.[30]

Initially concerned about the blood and saliva collections, I find that I barely notice them. The avalanche of images and feelings, both bright and dark, fills all mental space, leaving almost no room to perceive external interferences with the body. These samples will be crucial in the clinical trial of DMT, to shed some light on the obscure terrain where the mind's biochemistry secretes moods, traumas, ideas, and the will to live.

Or not.

The final procedures of the experiment I underwent at HUOL proceed without mishaps, without joy, without impatience, and without rapture. Once again, I notice a certain dullness and difficulty in understanding and filling out, at Falchi's request, the scales on the intensity and quality of the experience. The psychiatrist asks several times if I am feeling well. He informs me that everything went well with the pilot experiment, except for a few failures in the EEG data collection and blood draw, and releases me for lunch and to go home. My companion, Claudia, is already waiting. It's almost three in the afternoon, and I am once again surprised at how much time has passed. Lunch arrives in a lunchbox: fish with rice, beans, and vegetables. Claudia gets roast beef with rice, beans, and corn meal farofa. Feeling a bit nauseous, with a headache but hungry, I finish my plate and also Claudia's.

Back at the guesthouse, I feel an overwhelming need to go outside, see the sky, and walk, which I do for forty minutes. Sweat pours from my skin, accompanying the rush of emotions and thoughts that I later try to condense into a narrative for our hosts, which helps organize my ideas, though with the growing sense that reason is striving to fill gaps in what it cannot access. It feels almost like an imposture, a creative reconstruction driven by the desire to communicate to others an ineffable experience. I recall the seventh aphorism of the *Tractatus Logico-Philosophicus* by the Austrian philosopher Ludwig Wittgenstein: Whereof one cannot speak, thereof one must be silent.

The main residue is the powerful impact of the second dose. There is a suspicion that the experience might be too disturbing for someone without prior contact with psychedelics, which could trigger panic, as I doubt that such a borderline experience can always have therapeutic value, at least for those with severe depression.

Very little is still known about the mechanism behind the psychological benefit, Dráulio warns. It cannot be ruled out that the effect is mainly biochemical, which could even allow future psychedelic medications to be administered under sedation, to avoid potentially tumultuous trips. In the afternoon, at a meeting I did not attend, right after the double session, the team decided to reduce the subsequent doses to 15 mg and 60 mg, at least for some volunteers, Dráulio would later inform me (mine, in the pilot, had been 30 mg and 100 mg). I recommend they think carefully before adopting this change. After all, it may just be the scruple of someone inclined to caution, like me, who is not attracted to heroic journeys with psychedelics. In the end, I am not a depressed patient seeking a cure, but rather someone interested in the experience to anchor in vivid accounts the therapeutic potential envisioned by science, even if it brings self-knowledge and peace as a side effect—and nothing adverse, on the contrary, quite welcome.

My greatest surprise: realizing that inhaled DMT triggers intense, unsettling moments, but does not bring to consciousness contents (memories, people, traumas, events), as is common with the prolonged effect of ayahuasca. Thrown into a strange space, one may find it wondrous, but also inhospitable. If the hypothesis of the UFRN team is confirmed, this brief visit to the depths of the psyche provided by inhaled DMT may serve to bring some transcendent light even to those trapped in depression.[31]

A Team Committed to Bringing the Power of Jurema to the Public Health System

The chemist Sérgio Ruschi Bergamachi Silva, 31 years old at the time of our meeting,[32] had never even tasted alcohol, let alone DMT or any other consciousness-altering substance. He received a strict upbringing from his father, a military man from Monte Alegre, in the interior of Rio Grande do Norte, who was surprised when his son told him of his plan to analyze black jurema—in his view, a tree good only for fence posts and charcoal. Researching the psychedelic substance changed the son's view of drugs: "Psychoactive molecules are not what people make them out to be, nor what I learned all my life," he says. "DMT is a molecule like any other."

Ruschi completed his undergraduate degree at UFRN in 3.5 of the usual four years. In 2013, at age 22, he passed a competitive exam for the Federal Rural University of the Semi-Arid (UFERSA), in Mossoró (RN), 280 km from Natal. He commuted by bus to the capital, four hours each way, to attend classes for his master's at UFRN. His dissertation dealt with computer simulation of proteins and their molecular interaction with drugs—a lot of theory and programming, little hands-on laboratory work. Tired of so much travel, he managed to transfer as a UFERSA employee to UFRN in 2017. He saw an opportunity arise with an opening at the IC to operate a chromatograph, equipment used at the institute to identify the chemical composition of controlled substances.

The work plan in Dráulio's laboratory, in partnership with the company Biomind, included developing an optimized method to synthesize N,N-dimethyltryptamine with the requisites of green chemistry, aimed at producing fewer polluting residues. Ruschi joined the group with the mission of carrying out the project, assisted by undergraduate researcher Érica Pantrigo and tasked with improving the extraction and purification of DMT from jurema. The first batches supplied the initial experiments of the clinical trial on depression as well as animal studies.

The tree material, brought frozen by Dráulio from the Logradouro farm, is dried in an oven for 24 to 48 h. Once ground, the bark from each root yields 150 to 250 g of fine powder, the color of ground cinnamon, which is then treated with the solvent hexane. Separated from the aqueous phase in a separatory funnel, the hexane is evaporated under vacuum and recovered for reuse. From two hundred milliliters of solution, five milliliters remain, which are frozen for five to eight hours, after which DMT precipitates as crystals. With an average yield of 0.3%, 250 g of root powder can produce 750 mg of DMT. This is enough for twelve individual 60-mg doses used in the depression experiment.

Ruschi says he was surprised by the simplicity of the procedure. The real challenge, however, will be laboratory synthesis from scratch—or rather, from off-the-shelf chemical reagents, without using natural raw material, in order to produce larger quantities. To develop the process, he is collaborating with his former organic chemistry professor at UFRN, Fabrício Gava Menezes. The plan is to start with small amounts, 0.5 to five grams. Once the process is mastered, they will scale up to twenty grams, nearly thirty times more than what is obtained from root extraction. Menezes and Ruschi are also eager to innovate by making modifications to the DMT molecule to improve its efficacy. They will use computational models to seek suggestions for refining the biological and therapeutic effects, potentially increasing the antidepressant potential and making the experience smoother.

Sophie Laborde, 25, responsible for conducting integration sessions—conversations to evaluate the experience, as psychologists like her and psychiatrists like Falchi call it—is almost forty years younger than I am. Despite the age difference, the conversation about the volunteer's intimate feelings flows without barriers after the two DMT doses. A psychology graduate from UFRN, she is one of the few humanities scholars in Dráulio's natural sciences laboratory at the ICe. The clinical trial is the subject of her master's thesis.

Her interest in psychoactive substances began with her contact with ayahuasca during a difficult period in her life at age nineteen. Her father, a Frenchman living in Brazil, had been diagnosed with cancer in 2016 and had returned to live with the family from whom he had been estranged. After hearing accounts about the brew, she sought help in the Amazonian concoction and underwent one of the most significant experiences of her life. "I found a lot of understanding toward my father," she says. "Understanding and empathy, including for myself." She has had other experiences with DMT, with shamans and in sessions of the ayahuasca-based religion União do Vegetal.

She passed a competitive exam for a temporary position as a legal psychologist and worked for two years in conciliation processes. She spent the 2021 pandemic isolated in Pipa Beach, providing virtual psychotherapy sessions. She also accompanied groups of young people who used psychedelics, whether recreationally at parties or in search of self-knowledge, usually with urban neo-shamans. Most told her they had never had the chance to talk about these experiences, good or bad. In January 2022, she returned to Natal with plans to pursue a master's degree in France, which she had postponed due to the covid-19 pandemic. A colleague from her clinic then told her that Dráulio's group was looking for psychologists to conduct integration sessions with participants in the DMT trial. She applied for the position and began attending meetings, initially intimidated by the technical and medical terminology. She became enthusiastic, though, about the opportunity to do what she loves most: listening to people.

"If we can achieve the same results as ayahuasca [*obtained in the 2018 study by Dráulio's group*] with ten minutes of DMT, imagine the impact on public health. A drug that could greatly help those who currently have no help." She means help from available antidepressants, referring to the 30% or more of people with treatment-resistant depression. Laborde believes it is important for researchers and therapists—both women and men—to be familiar with the psychedelics they administer. Based on her own experience, she leans toward the hypothesis that something in the psychedelic journey itself contributes to the therapeutic benefit, not just the drug's biochemical impact, and that having gone through it makes listening less difficult. "For the volunteer [in the clinical trial], knowing that the researcher has taken and trusts the substance can be very reassuring." This is not a consensus among psychedelic researchers, as some advocate abstinence as a condition for detachment and objectivity.

The physiologist Nicole Galvão-Coelho has been collaborating with Dráulio for over a decade. She was responsible, for example, for the blood analyses of participants in the pioneering 2018 placebo-controlled ayahuasca study for depression. She also investigates the effects of the brew in marmosets isolated for nine weeks, during which they enter a state equivalent to human depression. She has been administering the beverage to them every three weeks, with an apparent prophylactic effect.[33]

In previous studies with ayahuasca, the effective dose of DMT was known only imprecisely. After all, the metabolism of the psychoactive compound varies greatly from individual to individual. With the substance being inhaled in a known quantity, the eleven successive blood samples allow for more precise determination of its concentration in the volunteer's body at each moment. This makes it possible to correlate these concentrations with scores from psychometric scales (questionnaires) used to measure the antidepressant response. The most complex aspect is collecting samples during the psychedelic effect, which ideally should not require the patient's attention, the researcher notes. DMT is a vasoconstrictor, which makes it difficult to access the vein, hence the use of a catheter rather than a needle. "Now there is a new challenge: to be very agile while also ensuring the volunteer's comfort." For this reason, needle phobia is among the exclusion criteria for the clinical trial conducted at the ICe and UFRN. The same applies to cardiac problems and a propensity for or history of psychosis, including in first-degree relatives, since the psychedelic compound from jurema, like other psychedelics, can trigger a psychotic episode.

The blood and saliva analyses will go beyond determining the concentration of DMT in the blood. In previous experiments, Galvão-Coelho had already been measuring biomarkers that the literature has associated with depressive disorder and antidepressant effects, such as cortisol, known as the stress hormone. Another factor under investigation is C-reactive protein, an indicator of inflammation, since the brains of people with depression are often inflamed (although it is not yet clear whether this is a result or a causal component of the disorder). Another is growth hormone (GH), which is involved in the response to acute stress and appears to be related to depression. Finally, the group's attention is focused on brain-derived neurotrophic factor (BDNF). This protein is found in significant amounts in the hippocampus and cerebral cortex and is involved in neuroplasticity, that is, the formation of connections between neurons and, through this process, in learning. One of the mechanisms proposed to explain the antidepressant effect of psychedelics points in this direction: they may facilitate the opening of new pathways in the mind, allowing individuals to escape the rumination that in some cases can lead to suicidal ideation.

The Onofre Lopes Hospital at UFRN, affiliated with the Brazilian health system SUS, provides between eight hundred and nine hundred psychiatric consultations per month, of which 10% to 20% are for patients with depression. Each week, between ten and twenty of these patients are diagnosed with the treatment-resistant form of the disorder—people who have tried two or more antidepressant medications without success. There will be no shortage of participants for the clinical trial in partnership with the ICe, reports Emerson Arcoverde Nunes. The psychiatrist, who was forty years old at the time of the interview in May 2022, also collaborated with Dráulio on the pioneering ayahuasca study.

The Northern neighborhoods of Natal, the physician explains, have about 400,000 residents and only one Psychosocial Care Center (CAPS), which is specialized in alcohol and drug abuse rather than mood disorders such as depression. "Everything falls to us," the psychiatrist complains. To make matters worse, with the prioritization of care for covid-infected patients in 2020–2021, the hospital saw its psychiatric beds reduced from 130 to 65. The public mental health service urgently needs alternative treatments, according to the physician. Arcoverde places great hope in DMT: "The more options, the better, and new options at that," he says. He cites the anesthetic ketamine, which has been used with some success against depression, but does not work for half of patients. "DMT has a strong and acute effect; it can pull someone out of suicidal ideation," the psychiatrist hopes. "The advantage of DMT is that it is a different medication, with different mechanisms of action and different contraindications," he argues. The most recent pharmacological innovations for depression emerged nearly half a century ago, with selective serotonin reuptake inhibitors, which act upon the neurotransmitter system also targeted by psychedelics.

Marcelo Falchi Parra Carvalho Silva, 32 years old, Arcoverde's colleague at the ICe and at the hospital, is also a psychiatrist. Originally from the town of Votuporanga (in the state of São Paulo), he was based in the city of Campinas until October 2021, where he worked with Luís Fernando Tófoli and Isabel Wießner on experiments investigating the effect of LSD on cognition.[34] He left everything behind and moved to Natal with just two suitcases, drawn by the opportunity to study DMT after being hired by the British company Biomind as head of the psychiatric research unit in Brazil. His fascination with the molecule is such that he has a tattoo of it on his back (his first, "impactful," experience with N,N-dimethyltryptamine occurred during his psychiatry residency). He worked in the SUS and began a master's degree at Unicamp, which he would obtain in 2024, but felt dissatisfied with the precariousness of procedures in his specialty. He wanted to better understand consciousness and its alteration under the influence of psychedelics, a process he calls "phenomenological mapping."

His main role in Natal is to work as a physician-scientist, he explains. "There [in Campinas] I had to work as a doctor in a SUS ward, prescribing treatments of limited efficacy, dedicating myself to science only secondarily." Falchi considers it unfeasible, within the SUS system, to implement a model similar to psychedelic-assisted psychotherapy as currently being investigated in the United States. In addition to being expensive, the monitoring of lengthy dosing sessions by two therapists opens the door to undue interference by professionals who are not highly trained, since the patient becomes suggestible: "It's a very wide window for the doctor to introduce undesirable elements, whether out of malice or lack of preparation," he worries (and, indeed, at least one case of sexual abuse by therapists was among the objections raised by the FDA in August 2024 to MDMA therapy for post-traumatic stress disorder).

Should shorter DMT sessions prove effective against depression, the psychiatrist from São Paulo envisions a different care model. For example, clinics specializing in administering psychedelic doses, monitoring patients during the procedure, and returning them to the psychological or psychiatric services where they were already being treated. The DMT would provide a burst of neuroplasticity, without the elaboration of content at the peak of the psychedelic experience, which is brief and intense. Only in the subsequent period, during subacute effects, would psychotherapeutic treatment in the strict sense take place. For this, it would be necessary to train far fewer therapists than in the usual psychedelic psychotherapy protocol, and the training could be shorter. "Because I come from the SUS, I know it won't work." For Lady gaga, maybe, not for Jane Doe.

Notes

1. The reports that gave rise to this chapter were originally published by *Folha de S.Paulo* in July 2022, in the series "A Ressurreição da Jurema," and can be found in Portuguese at: <https://www1.folha.uol.com.br/ilustrissima/2022/07/da-caatinga-ao-laboratorio-cientistas-investigam-efeito-antidepressivo-de-psicodelico.shtml> and <https://www1.folha.uol.com.br/ilustrissima/2022/07/reporter-conta-experiencia-de-inalar-dmt-psicodelico-em-teste-contra-depressao.shtml>

2. On August 9, 2024, the United States drug agency (FDA) rejected Lykos Therapeutics' application for licensing MDMA-assisted psychotherapy to treat PTSD and requested a new phase III clinical trial, in addition to the two already conducted by the company, to obtain new data demonstrating the efficacy and safety of the new treatment. The decision put the brakes on the wave of optimism surrounding psychedelic therapies and likely postponed, for several years, the return of these drugs to the pharmacopeia authorized for mental health. Expectations for approval by the FDA then shifted to phase III studies by the Usona Institute (Wisconsin, USA) and Compass Pathways (United Kingdom) with psilocybin for depression.

3. Marcelo Leite, "Brasil é o 3° país com mais artigos de impacto sobre psicodélicos." *Folha de S.Paulo*, Feb 9, 2021.

4. David Wyndham Lawrence, Bhanu Sharma, Roland R. Griffiths, and Robin Carhart-Harris, "Trends in Top-Cited Articles on Classic Psychedelics." *Journal of Psychoactive Drugs*, v. 53, no. 4, pp. 283–98, Feb. 3, 2021.

5. Dráulio B. de Araújo et al., "Seeing With the Eyes Shut: Neural Basis of Enhanced Imagery Following Ayahuasca Ingestion." *Human Brain Mapping*, v. 33, pp. 2550–60, Nov. 2012.

6. Sendi Reis Arruda, *Diversidade e Estrutura Genética de* Mimosa tenuiflora *(Wild.) Poir.: Importante recurso florestal do semiárido brasileiro.* Jequié, BA: UESB, 2014. pp. 16–7.

7. Ministry of the Environment, "Caatinga." Available at: <https://antigo.mma.gov.br/biomas/caatinga.html>. Accessed: Dec. 20, 2024.

8. MapBiomas, "Caatinga perde 160 mil ha de superfície de água e mais de 10% da vegetação nativa nos últimos 37 anos." Available at: <https://brasil.mapbiomas.org/2022/10/06/caatinga-perde-160-mil-ha-de-superficie-de-agua-e-mais-de-10-de-vegetacao-nativa-nos-ultimos-37-anos/>. Accessed: Dec. 20, 2024.

9. Sendi Reis Arruda, *Diversidade e Estrutura Genética de* Mimosa tenuiflora *(Wild.) Poir.: Importante recurso florestal do semiárido brasileiro.* Jequié, BA: UESB, 2014. p. 59.

10. José Otamar Falcão de Morais, *O Químico Oswaldo Gonçalves de Lima: Comentários sobre uma rica existência.* Recife: UFPE, n.d.

11. *Arquivos do Instituto de Pesquisas Agronômicas*, v. 4, pp. 45–80, 1946.

12. Oswaldo Gonçalves de Lima, *Goethe e a Química*. Recife: Editora UFPE, 1966. Available at: <https://editora.ufpe.br/books/catalog/book/323> . Accessed: Dec. 20, 2024.

13. Richard H. F. Manske, "A Synthesis of the Methyltryptamines and Some Derivatives." *Canadian Journal of Research*, v. 5, pp. 592–600, Nov. 1931. Available at: <https://cdnsciencepub.com/doi/10.1139/cjr31-097 >. Accessed: Dec. 20, 2024.

14. Stephen Szara, "Dimethyltryptamine: Its Metabolism in Man; the Relation of its Psychotic Effect to Serotonin Metabolism." *Experientia*, v. 12, pp. 441–2, Nov. 1956. Available at: <https://doi.org/10.1007/bf02157378>. Accessed: Dec. 20, 2024.

15. F. Benington, R. D. Morin, and L. C. Clark, Jr., "5-Methoxy-N,N -Dimethyltryptamine, A Possible Endogenous Psychotoxin." *Alabama Journal of Medical* Science, v. 2, no. 4, 1965. Available at: <https://archives.lib.purdue.edu/repositories/2/archival_objects/24515> . Accessed: Dec. 20, 2024.

16. Ann Shulgin and Alexander Shulgin, *T i HKAL: The Continuation.* Berkeley, CA: Transform Press, 2011, p. 248.

17. Ibid., pp. 246–68.

18. Richard Evans Schultes, Albert Hofmann and Christian Rätsch, *Plants of the Gods: Their Sacred, Healing, and Hallucinogenic Powers*, revised

and expanded edition. Rochester, VT: Healing Arts Press, 2001. pp. 138–9.

19. Pedro Luz, *Carta Psiconáutica*. Rio de Janeiro: Dantes, 2015. p. 222.

20. World Health Organization, "Depressive Disorder (depression)". March 31, 2023. Available at: <https://www.who.int/news-room/fact-sheets/detail/depression> . Accessed: December 20, 2024.

21. Marcelo Leite, "Ayahuasca diminui sintomas de depressão em pesquisa brasileira". *Folha de S.Paulo*, June 15, 2018.

22. Fernanda Palhano-Fontes et al., "Rapid Antidepressant Effects of the Psychedelic Ayahuasca in Treatment-Resistant Depression: A Randomized Placebo-Controlled Trial". *Psychological Medicine*, v. 49, n. 4, pp. 655–63, March 2019.

23. Kim van Oorsouw et al., "Therapeutic Effect of an Ayahuasca Analogue in Clinically Depressed Patients: a Longitudinal Observational Study". *Psychopharmacology*, v. 239, pp. 1839–52, January 24, 2022. Available at: <https://doi.org/10.1007/s00213-021-06046-9> . Accessed: December 20, 2024.

24. Marcelo Leite, "Faltam estudos maiores e melhores para consagrar psicodélicos". Virada Psicodélica. *Folha de S.Paulo*, June 28, 2022. Available at: <https://www1.folha.uol.com.br/blogs/virada-psicod elica/2022/06/faltam-estudos-maiores-e-melhores-para-consagrar-psi codelicos.shtml> . Accessed: December 20, 2024.

25. Elisaldo A. Carlini and Lucas O. Maia, "Plant and Fungal Hallucinogens as Toxic and Therapeutic Agents", in P. Gopalakrishnakone, Célia Regina Carlini and Rodrigo Ligabue-Braun (eds.), *Plant Toxins*. Dordrecht: Springer, 2019. p. 7.

26. Marcelo Falchi-Carvalho et al., "Safety and Tolerability of Inhaled N,N -Dimethyltryptamine (BMND01 candidate): a Phase 1 Clinical Trial". *European Neuropsychopharmacology*, v. 80, pp. 27–35, March 2024. Available at: <https://doi.org/10.1016/j.euroneuro.2023.12.006> . Accessed: December 20, 2024.

27. Marcelo Leite, "UFRN recupera jurema em artigo sobre uso seguro de DMT inalada". Virada Psicodélica. *Folha de S.Paulo*, December 28, 2023. Available at: <https://www1.folha.uol.com.br/blogs/virada-psi codelica/2023/12/ufrn-recupera-jurema-em-artigo-sobre-uso-seguro-de-dmt-inalada.shtml> . Accessed on: December 20, 2024.

28. Marcelo Leite, "Ano começa movimentado para a medicina psicodélica." Virada Psicodélica. *Folha de S.Paulo*, January 8, 2024.

Available at: <https://www1.folha.uol.com.br/blogs/virada-psicod elica/2024/01/ano-2024-comecou-movimentado-para-a-medicina-psi codelica.shtml> . Accessed on: December 20, 2024.

29. Deepak Cyril D'Souza et al., "Exploratory Study of the Dose-Related Safety, Tolerability, and Efficacy of Dimethyltryptamine (DMT) in Healthy Volunteers and Major Depressive Disorder." *Neuropsychophar-macology*, v. 47, pp. 1854–62, Sept. 2022. Available at: <https://doi.org/10.1038/s41386-022-01344-y>. Accessed on: December 20, 2024.

30. Johannes T. Reckweg et al., "A Phase 1/2 Trial to Assess Safety and Effi-cacy of a Vaporized 5-Methoxy- N,N -Dimethyltryptamine Formu-lation (GH 001) in Patients with Treatment-Resistant Depression." *Frontiers in Psychiatry*, v. 14, June 20, 2023. Available at: <https://doi.org/10.3389/fpsyt.2023.1133414> . Accessed on: December 20, 2024.

31. Richard J. Zeifman et al., "Preliminary Evidence for the Importance of Therapeutic Alliance in MDMA -Assisted Psychotherapy for Posttrau-matic Disorder." *European Journal of Psychotraumatology*, v. 15, January 4, 2024. Available at: <https://doi.org/10.1080/20008066.2023.229 7536> . Accessed on: December 20, 2024.

32. Interview conducted on May 18, 2022.

33. Maria Lara Porpino de Meiroz Grilo et al., "Prophylactic Action of Ayahuasca in a Non-Human Primate Model of Depressive-Like Behavior." *Frontiers in Behavioral Science*, v. 16, November 4, 2022. Available at: <https://www.frontiersin.org/articles/10.3389/fnbeh.2022.901425/full> . Accessed on: December 20, 2024.

34. Isis M. Ornelas et al., "Nootropic Effects of LSD: Behavioral, Molecular and Computational Evidence." *Experimental Neurology*, v. 356, October 2022. Available at: <https://doi.org/10.1016/j.expneu rol.2022.114148> . Accessed on: December 20, 2024.

The Origin of Catimbó in Alhandra, a Former Colonial Settlement

There is a profusion of entities in the Jurema Sagrada that might leave readers as disoriented as I was during my first encounter with the Jurema of Alhandra (state of Paraíba), a confusion gradually clarified by the work of anthropologists such as Clarice Mota, Luiz Assunção, Rodrigo Grünewald, and Sandro de Salles. Although it encompasses many variations—the religiosity that emerged in the Northeast, after all, springs from the newest sap rising from the rhizomatic roots of Catimbó, a result of the adaptability of Brazilian Indigenous peoples under colonial rule—the Jurema Sagrada presents, in various places, something close to a doctrinal core with its own pantheon of deified beings.

"Jurema," to begin with, encompasses a multiplicity of meanings, what Clarice Mota called the "Jurema complex": it is the tree from which the ritual beverage is prepared, generally the black jurema (jurema-preta, in Portuguese) though other varieties recognized by popular tradition are also used (jurema-branca, jurema-de-caboclo, jurema-de-espinho, jurema-das-matas, and jureminha); in places of worship where none of these trees are present, or in ritual halls, it is almost always represented by a "tronqueira" (a piece of wood symbolizing the sacred plant); it is the beverage itself, or entheogen, the "wine of jurema" prepared from the root or bark of the plant; a mythical Indigenous woman, transfigured into the entity Cabocla Jurema, who would later become prominent in the Afro-Brazilian rituals of Umbanda; and, finally, it lends its name to the very religion that continues the tradition of Catimbó, the Jurema Sagrada.

As anthropologist Rodrigo Grünewald noted when commenting on Marcos Albuquerque's fieldwork at the Terreiro de Umbanda Oxum Taladami

© The Author(s), under exclusive license to Springer Nature Switzerland AG 2026
M. Leite, *The Psychedelic Science of the Jurema Tree*, Copernicus Books, https://doi.org/10.1007/978-3-032-22705-8_2

in Campina Grande (Paraíba), there would be no Jurema Sagrada without the influence of Christianity, which sanctified even the plant itself, venerated by Indigenous people, catimbozeiros, and juremeiros: "It is in the jurema wood [...] that the spirits are settled, since it would contain the presence of God, for Jesus is said to have wet the jurema with his blood when he leaned against it while hiding from Roman persecution with Herod," he says. This myth is retold in various ways in different places. "What matters is the general idea that the blood of Jesus gave the plant the sacred power of communion with God."[1] On a Jurema table (or shrine), maracás, or master rattles—traditionally made from round gourds called cuité—are indispensable; as are pipes, or marcas, used to blow purifying smoke through the mouthpiece; and the princesas, originally clay vessels for holding and drinking the jurema beverage, now a name given to glass goblets and cups filled with water. The first two, maracás and smoke, are the most representative elements of Indigenous origin, already recorded by missionaries in accounts of the so-called heresies at the beginning of the colonial era. "The smoke, cast as a blessing, a powerful exorcism, a 'permanent' feature in Catimbó, is linked to Indigenous liturgy, observed in the sixteenth and seventeenth centuries," noted folklorist Luís da Câmara Cascudo.[2] To these were added objects and symbols incorporated through syncretism with European magical practices, such as keys and six-pointed stars, the sign or seal of Solomon, which in the local vernacular became known as "sino Salamão"—and it is not surprising to also find a small bell on the table ("sino" in Portuguese means bell).

The central entities of Jurema are the masters, as the sorcerers of seventeenth-century Portugal were also called, according to Mário de Andrade.[3] Among practitioners of the Jurema Sagrada, the title refers both to juremeiros of great stature, holders of "science" in life, and to those who, upon "disincarnating," come to occupy a higher plane sometimes referred to as the "astral," under the influence of Kardecism. There, they live in villages or cities, each inhabited or led by three masters, and twelve of these make up a State, or Kingdom. From this other plane, the enchanted masters and mistresses come down to "work," i.e., perform healings, give advice, or make and break spells, once incorporated or manifested in mediums, vessels, or "irradiated" persons. When they descend, the masters usually adopt characteristic postures, manners, or adornments that allow for identification by the initiated; they also request cachaça (sugarcane brandy), jurema, a pipe or cigar, and give "messages" (advice) or recommend herbs, medicinal infusions, syrups (lambedores, generally sweetened with honey), baths, prayers, offerings, and obligations. Among the most revered is Mestre Carlos, who cleansed Mário de Andrade and has several songs dedicated to him, such as this one recorded by the folklorist and musicologist:

Mestre Carlos is a good master
Who learned without being taught
He lay fallen for three days
At the root of the Jurema tree
When he rose up
He was ready to work
Triumphing at the hidden table
At his own table, he laughed
   (All quotations in this chapter were translated by the author with the help of artificial intelligence)

According to José Ribeiro, in *Catimbó, Magia do Nordeste*,[4] Mestre Carlos, sung in some Jurema traditions as the King of Masters, was the son of a famous catimbozeiro, Mestre Inácio de Oliveira. A mischievous boy, by the age of thirteen (other versions say twelve) he already enjoyed drinking and gambling, much to his father's dismay. Escaping supervision, Carlos managed to enter the room where Catimbó rituals were held, took ritual instruments, and went out into the field, determined to open a table (perform a ritual) by himself far from home, at the foot of a jurema tree. "Not knowing how to close the session, he was taken by the masters and died. Three days later, his half-decayed body was found," Ribeiro records. Very popular, Mestre Carlos displays a strong personality when he incorporates into a medium: he is jealous, asks for alcoholic drinks, becomes cross-eyed, and puckers his mouth, speaking with great fluency. He is attributed with great powers, for both good and evil; he is one of the most popular masters.

Mário de Andrade considered the story of Mestre Carlos beautiful and impressive. "From a very young age, he proved to be an exceptional boy. As mischievous as the Devil, he mingled with fallen women and other very free people," he records in *O Turista Aprendiz*. "His father, Inácio de Oliveira, a catimbozeiro, was disappointed in his son, and did not want to initiate him into witchcraft."[5]

Mestre Germano, João Germano das Neves, the "devotee of Xaramundi," was the one who performed the body-closing ritual for the São Paulo native during his 1928 visit to Natal, according to Câmara Cascudo.[6] Before passing away, Xaramundi was a tuxaua (indigenous chief) in the Amazon forest, demonstrating great versatility as a healer. According to Ribeiro, one of his specialties is cleansing, the power to remove impurities from a person's body or to undo a spell. He is himself a sorcerer, avenger, and protector. One of his songs says:

> *By the trunk I climbed and by the branches I descended,*
> *By the sound of my flute I went,*
> *By the sound of my flute I came…*
> *I am Mestre Xaramundi! I am Mestre Xaramundi!*
> *I am from the trunk of the Jurema, I am the Healing Master!*[7]

Mário de Andrade describes in some detail his experience of the body-closing ritual with the help of Xaramundi in the backyard of Dona Plastina, in the Redinha neighborhood of Natal, on December 28, 1928. Several masters were incorporated by the mediums Manuel, with *pince-nez*, and the mulatto João: the hero Felipe Camarão and the beautiful Nanã-Giê; Agicé and Manicoré; and Xaramundi himself, who resolved the mediums' difficulties by incorporating into João and finally opening the table. But it was Mestre Carlos, according to Andrade, the "flower of the night," who truly led the ritual:

> […] the "one who learned without being taught," with his twelve demateri-alized years, a Pernambucano son of an Amazonian, mischievous and playful, the only master allowed to laugh during the sessions, Mestre Carlos is the one who protects, at all hours of every day, the Brazilian who now writes to you.[8]

Mário de Andrade so characterized the experience at Dona Plastina's house: "It is impossible to describe everything that took place in that ceremony absurd, a mixture of sincerity and charlatanism, ridiculous, religious, comic, dramatic, unnerving, repugnant, deeply moving, all blended together. And poetic." Mário goes on to say that, despite the ridicule he subjected himself to out of mere curiosity, the repugnance did not linger in his memory; instead, he felt "overtaken by lyricism before those endless songs, heard in their natural setting."[9]

The memory imbued with lyricism, however, did not prevent the São Paulo scholar from recounting, in a jocular tone later on, his escape at the end of the session:

> And so I left Dona Plastina's little house, quite lyrical and in the mood to laugh, treading the shifting sand as I fled in search of a car that awaited me at a distance, on solid ground. The darkness was complete because the Moon had already gone to rest. But nothing happened to me. I reached the car easily, and it took me to where my friends were already waiting, somewhat anxious. I did not slip on the sand, I did not break my leg, no dog barked at me, there were no bandits in Natal, because my body, by the musical power of the gods, was forever shielded against the injuries of the air, the earth, the underworld, and the waters of the sea. Price: thirty thousand réis.[10]

Álvaro Carlini, who examined the material collected and recorded by the 1938 Folklore Mission organized by Andrade, listed the names of several masters, caboclos, and kings venerated in Jurema: Antônia, Filomena, Leonor, Maria de Luanda, Sebastiana, Caboco Tupi, Chocolate, Arruda, Francisco Velho, Heraqueto, Jandaraí, João Cigano, José da Cruz, José de Arruda, José Severino, Luís Inácio, Major do Dia, Malunguinho, Maraú, Mariano, Odilon, Penduarana, and Periquitinho.[11]

The most well-known is perhaps Zé Pelintra, or Seu Zé, generally depicted as a Black trickster from Rio de Janeiro in a white suit, an evolved spirit who, according to some Jurema practitioners, no longer possesses mediums and occupies a central place in a phalanx of Zés: Zé de Santana, Zé Menino, Zé Boiadeiro, Zé Bebim.[12] "For many, Zé Pelintra would be José de Aguiar, who is said to have been born in 1813 and died at the age of 114," writes Sandro de Salles.[13] Luiz Antonio Simas provides, in *Umbandas: Uma História do Brasil*, the most extensive biography of Seu Zé, who is said to have been born in Cabo de Santo Agostinho (Pernambuco), grown up in Afogados da Ingazeira, and lived in Recife, on Rua da Amargura, near the bohemian district. Hopelessly in love with Maria Luziara, one of the women who made a living on Rua da Guia and who herself would become a famous Jurema entity, Zé set out on a journey through the Northeast and was initiated into the Sacred Jurema rites by Master Inácio, who is said to have acquired his knowledge from the Caeté indigenous people.

These travels took him to Rio de Janeiro, where he ultimately merged with the figure of the typical malandro of Rio's macumba, living in Lapa and dying in a fight in Santa Teresa, as Simas recounts: "He abandoned the garb of a Jurema master and appears in the terreiros of Guanabara as a refined trickster, dressed in a white linen suit, chrome shoes, Panama hat, and red tie."[14] Elsewhere, he is described with a cane and pipe, a long white or checkered shirt, white trousers rolled up at the legs, a red scarf around his neck, and always barefoot.

The female counterpart of the leading entities in circles of malandragem and exu gatherings are the pombajiras (or pombagiras), a word whose etymology Simas asserts certainly derives from the Angolan-Congolese cults of the inquices (divinities roughly corresponding to the orixás). One manifestation of the power of the streets in Central African cultures, he explains, is the inquice Bombojiro, "the feminine side of Aluvaiá, Mavambo, the lord of the crossroads, similar to the Yoruba Exu and the Fon vodum Elegbara."[15]

Reginaldo Prandi concurs that pombajira is a corruption of Bongbo-girá, the name of Exu in Angolan candomblé, from the Bantu tradition. In Umbanda, the sociologist of religions writes in *Brasil Africano*, "it is the spirit of a woman (not an orixá) who in life is said to have been a prostitute or courtesan, a woman of low moral standards, capable of dominating men through their sexual prowess, lovers of luxury, money, and all kinds of pleasures."[16] Highly sought after to resolve failures in love and sex, pombajiras are as outspoken and shameless as Exu, usually dressing in provocative and luxurious red and black clothing. There is a vast legion of pombajiras in Umbanda and, by extension, in Jurema Sagrada: Rainha, Sete Saias, Maria Molambo, Calunga, Cigana, do Cruzeiro, Cigana dos Sete Cruzeiros, das Almas, Maria Quitéria, Dama da Noite, Menina, Mirongueira, and Menina da Praia, among others.

One of the most famous pombajiras is Maria Padilha, who is said to have lived in fourteenth-century Seville, Spain, becoming the lover and advisor of King Peter I of Castile. According to Prandi, she is "the spirit of a very beautiful, white, seductive woman, who in life is said to have been a high-class prostitute or influential courtesan."[17] The sociologist cites the writer Marlyse Meyer, who in her book *Maria Padilha e toda sua quadrilha* traced the trajectory of this "imaginary avatar" from Montalvan to Beja, from Beja to Angola, from Angola to Recife, and from Recife to the terreiros throughout Brazil. According to Pai Rodney de Oxóssi, anthropologist, writer, and babalorixá, she reigns supreme at the crossroads, fostering meetings and partings, helping men and women along the obscure and uncertain paths of the heart: "She wins disputes, she retrieves a needle from the bottom of the sea," he wrote in his column for the magazine *Carta Capital*.[18] But he warns that it is wise not to meddle with Maria Padilha, a dangerous figure, as can be inferred from this excerpt:

> *They swore to kill me*
> *At the door of a cabaret*
> *They swore to kill me*
> *At the door of a cabaret*
> *I pass by in the day*
> *I pass by at night*
> *They don't kill me because they don't want to*

The pelintra and pombagira bodies function as antinomies to the colonizing project, notes Simas in *Umbandas*. "They escape normativity through trance, challenge canonical status in their swagger and performative narratives, and push to the limit a civilizing project that cannot cope with such radical otherness."

The caboclos and caboclas form a separate legion: that of the spirits of mythical Indigenous people who link Jurema to Brazilian soil and anchor its roots in an ancestral past that is renewed in the present. The caboclos, unlike the masters, are not associated with a historical time. Their origin is unknown and, in most cases, they appear as non-individualized entities, being identified by the name of their phalanx or tribe—Tupi, Tupinambá, Tabajara, explains the anthropologist Sandro de Salles.[19] Others are effigies of generic Indigenous figures, such as caboclos Pena Branca, Pena Vermelha, Pena Amarela, Pena Azul, Pena Preta ("pena" means feather in Portuguese)… Salles describes the incorporation of caboclos as often accompanied by spasms and convulsions, with the tip of the index finger pointed, representing the tip of an arrow: When they are not dancing, it is common to see them pacing restlessly from one side of the hall to the other, always serious, stern.[20]

Within the colonial-inspired hierarchy—and despite fulfilling the noble function of connecting with the ancestral roots of the land—according to some versions, caboclos are positioned below the masters in the Jurema pantheon. They are fierce, less developed entities, still in need of the doctrinal guidance and rationality present in the more evolved religiosity of Europe, now Spiritism, just as in the past heretics needed Jesuits and other priests to find the right spiritual path.

It is true that not everyone agrees with this subordination of caboclos to masters. The Jurema scholar Alexandre L'Omi L'Odó, for example, places the former above the latter, just below Tupã, Our Lady of the Conception, Jurema, and the Kings. Anthropologist Clélia Moreira Pinto concurs, for whom the caboclo is characterized as a higher entity than the master, being a "spirit of light" on a more advanced spiritual scale.[21] Anthropologist Luiz Assunção states that the caboclo evokes the idea of a colonized Indian, involved with the dominant white society and as the result of the intermingling of different ethnicities.[22] According to Francelino de Shapanan (or Xapanã), from the Casa das Minas de Toya Jarina in Diadema (state of São Paulo), the origin of the caboclo and the masters of Jurema lies in the indigenous people of the deep forest, the dense woods, but they must be disciplined: The Indian would be the beginning of the medium's indoctrination when he is just starting out and cannot yet distinguish between the terreiro and the forest, which is why he comes fierce, rough, undisciplined.[23] As can be seen even in doctrines where indigenous peoples appear as a kind of deity, the reach of prejudiced and demeaning notions associated with them is extensive.

Once disciplined and admitted into the jurema pantheon, the caboclos remain subordinate to the master spirits, as summarized by Luiz Antonio Simas and Luiz Rufino in *Fogo no Mato*: these masters were people who, in life, developed skills in the use of healing herbs and, after death, came to inhabit one of the mystical realms of Jurema. There, they are assisted by the Caboclos of Jurema, spirits of indigenous people who, in life, mastered the arts of war and healing.[24]

With all the plasticity inherited from indigenous cults, and especially through reciprocal influence with Umbanda, Jurema gradually incorporated other figures into its populous pantheon: old black men and women, gypsies, cowboys, and sailors. Perhaps the most peculiar, occupying a separate mythical category, are the Kings. There are the Europeanized King Solomon (frequently invoked at the opening of ceremonies),[25] King Heron and the King of Turkey, and others more obscure such as King Tanaruê. Noteworthy are Malunguinho and Canindé, sometimes referred to with an almost enigmatic plural title, Kings Malunguinho and Kings Canindé: according to L'Omi L'Odó, they were heroes in life recognized as a spiritual collective, as in the case of Malunguinho, a title designating a lineage of leaders of the Catucá Quilombo (campments of enslaved fugitives), the last of whom was killed in December 1835.[26]

"Malungo," a word of African origin with controversial etymology, means companion, comrade. In its diminutive form, it became a kind of title for the military chief of the Catucá Quilombo, which is said to have begun forming in 1824, according to records by Frei Caneca.[27] The chief Malunguinho had his headquarters at the Macacos site and extended his influence over several settlements in the Catucá forests. As one of the sixteen commanders died, the title passed to the next, according to L'Omi L'Odó. The first "king" of the quilombo, whose given name is unknown, is said to have been assassinated in 1829, after the government of the province of Pernambuco offered a reward of 100,000 réis for his head. The last, João Batista, died in 1835, according to a record from September of that year.

When it is sung in Jurema chants that "Malunguinho is Kings," says L'Omi L'Odó, head of the Casa das Matas do Reis Malunguinho in Recife, it is not a grammatical error made by the poor and uneducated people of Jurema, as members of the white elite, so zealous of their plurals and singulars, generally assume, but rather a deliberate reference to that collective title which, in the revered name, encapsulates the bravery and resistance of many rebellious Black people:

> *Malunguinho is in the forest,*
> *He is kings of the forest, he is Malunguinho!*
> *Close the door and listen to the forest,*
> *Set the watch on the path!*
> *Malunguinho is kings of the forest,*
> *He is kings of the forest, he is Malunguinho!*

Close the door, Malunguinho,
Block the neighbor's view!
Malunguinho is kings of the forest,
He is kings of the forest, he is Malunguinho!
Close the door and listen to the forest,
And close the neighbor's ears![28]

The multiple nature of the deity Malunguinho is also manifested in what L'Omi L'Odó describes as his quadruplicity: within Jurema, he is the only entity to simultaneously appear as caboclo, master, trunqueiro (trickster, Exu), and king, each represented in different statuettes, usually made of plaster. The Caboclo Malunguinho is depicted as an Indigenous man with a feathered headdress, a knife at his belt, red trousers, a necklace of teeth, a golden crown in his right hand, and a seven-pointed star in his left. The master appears as a Black man with trousers rolled up to the knee, holding a glass and a bottle, barefoot, with a jurema trunk between his legs. The trunqueiro may be portrayed as a Black boy sitting, arms wrapped around his legs, waiting for something at a crossroads. The king takes the form of a Moorish prince, with dark skin, wearing a vest, black boots, and a sword at his waist, a golden chalice in his right hand and a silver bottle in his left.[29]

A similar phenomenon occurs with another Jurema deity, Reis Canindé, a mythical figure of leadership in the Confederation of the Cariris, an Indigenous uprising against the Portuguese at the end of the seventeenth century, known as the War of the Barbarians. Also called by the Portuguese the King of the Janduís, Canindé died in 1699 in the Guaraíras settlement, now in Rio Grande do Norte, as recorded by Sandro Guimarães de Salles: "The centrality of these entities in the context of Jurema in Pernambuco and Paraíba highlights the impact these leaders had on humble people, whom they represented." The historical figures of Malunguinho and Canindé, the anthropologist notes, would have remained forgotten in public archives if not for the juremeiros who kept them alive and active as kings.[30]

The enchanted world of Jesus and Jurema, inhabited by entities such as caboclos and masters, is divided into kingdoms whose composition may vary from region to region, from one terreiro to another, and for this reason, they have been compiled into various lists by different authors. Câmara Cascudo, for example, lists seven of them (Vajucá, Tigre, Canindé, Urubá, Juremal, Fundo do Mar, and Josafá) and then another version with five (Vajucá, Juremal, Tanema, Urubá, and Josafá), attributing the two sets to different sources.[31] Mário de Andrade mentions eleven kingdoms: Juremal, Vajucá, Ondina, Rio Verde, Fundo do Mar, Cova de Salamão, Cidade Santa, Florestas Virgens, Vento, Sol, and Urubá.[32] Luiz Assunção cites several mystical places listed by Oneyda Alvarenga based on Catimbó songs collected by the 1938 Folklore Mission: Juremal, Cidade da Jurema, Torre da Jurema, Bom-Floral, Luanda, Maraú, Quatro Cidades, Cidade dos Pássaros, Vaucá, Vaiucá, Arubá, Bom-Passar, and Poço-Fundo.[33] At times, these mythical places are described as cities, as recorded by Sandro de Salles: Vajucá, Junça, Catucá, Manacá, Angico, Aroeira, and Jurema or Juremal[34] (all of the seven last names refer to plants; in addition, Catucá also refers to the central quilombo in Jurema mythology). L'Omi L'Odó provides a similar list to that of Salles, identifying plants for each designation: jurema (*Mimosa tenuiflora*), angico (*Anadenanthera colubrina*), junço (*Juncus effusus*),[35] jucá, vajucá or ajucá (*Caesalpinia ferrea*), manacá (*Tibouchina mutabilis*), catucá (*Salzmannia nitida*),[36] and aroeira (*Schinus terebinthifolius*).

Trees and herbs, as can be seen, are a central element in this religiosity with a strong Indigenous character, granting the black jurema of the Caatinga and the white jurema of the Zona da Mata—both small trees—a prominence comparable to that of the mighty sumaúma (*Ceiba pentandra*), which can exceed fifty meters in height and is venerated by some Amazonian peoples as the mother of nature and a privileged site for communication with ancestors. L'Omi L'Odó states the belief that the Indigenous religious tradition inherited by the juremeiros refers to the healing potential of trees and plants, as a recognition of their natural powers and also their psychoactive potentials. According to the self-baptized juremologist, manacá, aroeira, black jurema itself, junça, and jucá contain chemical compounds that may contribute to inducing trance in humans.[37]

When consecrated to a master, the jurema trees are called "cities"—for example, the city of Mestre Carlos. A commonly heard explanation holds that Jurema masters regarded as sorcerers, upon dying, could not be buried in Catholic cemeteries and ended up interred at the foot of one of these trees, becoming identified with it. An important city is said to have been swallowed by the sea at Tambaba beach, near Alhandra, a sacred site for the Jurema Sagrada, though better known to tourists as a nudist reserve. On the beach, there is a stretch where the cliffs recede from the sea, forming a kind of enclave among the rocks called the Portal da Encantaria, where a large cross is venerated by juremeiros, facing a rock in the sea, the Pedra de Xangô, which is said to emit a thunderous sound whenever a master dies.

From Acais to the Spiritist Center, the Survival of Masters and Caboclos

Since I began, in 2020, my research to understand black jurema and the virtually unknown religiosity that developed around it in the Northeast, it became clear that a visit to Alhandra would be essential. The city, near the southern coast of Paraíba, is unanimously regarded by all branches of juremeiros as the birthplace of the religion persecuted since colonial times that became known in the twentieth century as Catimbó. What in previous centuries were varied and scattered religious practices found in this city a more organized expression, with its own genealogy and monuments attesting that Amerindian rituals, blended with African and European elements, left deep roots in Northeastern Brazil's religious culture. The city itself arose on the ruins of an old indigenous settlement, when the land was divided and titled to descendants of the original peoples present there. At the center of the Catimbó origin myth—or its history, as seems more accurate—is a woman with family ties to this heritage, Maria do Acais, who lived on the property that bears her name and, upon her death, became the most celebrated of the Jurema masters.

Little remains of the old Acais estate, considered by many the seat of the Jurema Sagrada, except for the famous little church, a chapel with three narrow doors dedicated to Saint John the Baptist on the edge of highway PB-034, a stretch of the old Recife–João Pessoa road before the existence of BR-101. Next to the chapel stands a tree with round yellow flowers and brown pods, a jurema-de-mestre. Behind the building is a cement sculpture representing a stump of cut jurema-preta, marking the tomb of Mestre Flósculo Guimarães, son of Maria do Acais, who died in 1959. A few meters away, on the roadside, is a memorial dedicated to Mestre Zezinho, a renowned juremeiro who is said to have died there, run over after drinking cachaça at the Casa de Sete Portas, a still-standing warehouse not far away. On the edge of the asphalt, the low-roofed shelter built in his memory holds various offerings, mostly bottles of cachaça and candles, along with some flowers.

The main house of the estate, which stood on the other side of the highway, was demolished in 2008. The owner at the time, anticipating the completion of the listing process by the Institute of Historical and Artistic Heritage of the State of Paraíba (IPHAEP), ordered its demolition and the removal of the jurema "cities," trees consecrated to deceased masters. Maria Eugênia Gonçalves Guimarães, the second Maria do Acais, had lived there; she inherited the property in 1908 from her aunt, Maria Gonçalves de Barros, the first, both renowned and feared catimbozeiras, but it was the second who gave Acais, and Alhandra, their reputation as the cradle of the Jurema Sagrada.

Her granddaughter, Maria das Dores da Silva Guimarães, in an interview with anthropologist Rodrigo de Azeredo Grünewald,[38] attributed to the last Maria do Acais, who died in 1937, the introduction of "white table" rituals into the Catimbó cult. Previously, rites were performed on a cloth spread on the ground, preferably in the forest, under a jurema tree. The table may have been influenced by Kardecist Spiritism, which spread through Brazilian urban centers in the nineteenth and twentieth centuries, and with which the catimbozeira likely came into contact, probably while still living in Recife, where she was known as Maroca Feiticeira (something like Molly Witch). She moved to Alhandra around 1910, after her aunt died and left her the estate, but her connection to the city that arose from the Aratagui indigenous settlement was much older.

This last Maria do Acais was the daughter of Inácio Gonçalves de Barros, brother of Maria Gonçalves de Barros—the first—who served in the region as the last regent of the indigenous survivors of the Aratagui village. The first records of this Jesuit settlement date back to the 1590s, which would be elevated to the status of a town in 1765, following the Pombaline project to secularize and integrate indigenous settlements initiated with the creation of the Directorate of the Indians in 1757. The Portuguese Crown directive to name settlements after Portuguese cities was followed—in this case, Alhandra. In the early decades of the nineteenth century, the town had "two hundred hearths" (houses, or families), according to a record by vicar Braz de Melo in 1826, who described the inhabitants as idle, living off crabbing in the mangroves, with few dedicated to agriculture.[39] In the 2022 Brazilian Census, the city had 21,713 inhabitants.

In 1862, the emperor ordered the dissolution of the indigenous settlements in the province of Paraíba and the distribution of the land in plots to the indigenous people who were then concentrated in Baía da Traição and Alhandra. To carry out this task in the latter town, engineer Antônio Gonçalves da Justa Araújo was appointed, who demarcated plots of 62,500 square braças (approximately thirty hectares); the only exception was the plot marked out at twice the size for João Baptista Acais, who would lend his name to the renowned estate. Engineer Araújo recorded in his documents the dissatisfaction of Regent Mestre Inácio with the small size of the plots and with the non-indigenous settlers who were beginning to take them over. Regarding the partitioning of the territory, anthropologist Sandro de Salles noted that the indigenous people were gradually diluted among the poor free men, becoming part of the mass of small farmers—caboclos, Black people, mixed-race individuals, subjects of a silenced history, who would write the next chapters in the history of Jurema.

The poor people of the Northeast, without access to health clinics, pharmacies, or hospitals, ignored or mistreated by the Church, the Police, and the Justice system, have always turned to prayer healers and jurema practitioners to address their daily afflictions. In consultation sessions, often paid, they received from the masters and caboclos advice, divinations, or prescriptions for treatments for their ailments, such as herbal infusions, smoke cleansings, and herbal baths. The catimbozeiro was the doctor for humble, isolated people, not attended by the city doctors, says Sandro de Salles.[40]

Maria do Acais herself gained her reputation in this way, receiving not only the poor but also wealthy individuals from other cities, from João Pessoa to Recife. As early as 1938, the year after the juremeira's death, Gonçalves Fernandes (cited by Salles) noted that Maria do Acais enjoyed considerable prestige that established her reputation as a great catimbozeira. From Pernambuco to the state of Paraíba, people of all kinds came there to pay good money for the desired service. Seventy-two years later, after his field research in Alhandra, Salles himself found that the services provided by jurema practitioners were still in demand. Heirs to the tradition of the pajés, true healers, the juremeiros are knowledgeable in the secrets of herbs and roots, he explains. Unlike doctors, the masters know how to identify whether an illness is of the body or the spirit.

Raquel Néri de Freitas, Dona Raquel, who accompanied me on visits to the memorials of Flósculo and Zezinho and to the little church of Acais, is an heir to this tradition of healers. Next to her house in Alhandra, she runs a small shop with supplies for Sacred Jurema rituals, such as herbs, pipes, maracás, statuettes, tobacco, pembas (thick colored chalk sticks used to draw Umbanda symbols on the ground), and colored candles for saints not found in the city, where only white ones are sold. But it is far from there that she receives visitors and entities, at the Cantinho dos Benzedores (Prayers' Corner), a small farm acquired a few years ago in the rural neighborhood of Estiva—a region where Mestre Inácio, father of Maria do Acais 2, received his plot in the 1860s by order of Brazil's Emperor Dom Pedro II.

Tall and upright at 67 years old, at the time of my visit to her Cantinho (December 2022), Dona Raquel had just suffered a heart attack when she acquired the property. She says she was given three months to live, and buying land was the last thing on her mind. Her widow's pension barely covered the cost of her medication. She gave consultations from the shop, charging no one. In a trance, the entity she incorporated told her she would need to find another place for her work, "with an entrance and an exit." Upon returning from the hospital, her sister told her that a distressed man named Manuel had come to the shop, wanting to sell a plot of land at a very low price. Dona Raquel says she again felt the presence of the entity, now telling her: "It's mine." She sold another small plot and bought the farm.

Before that, she performed some rituals at a gongá (site for Afro-Brazilian worship) she maintained not far from there, which had belonged to the famous Mestra Aderita, but her descendants were increasingly uninterested in its upkeep, and she abandoned it. The newly acquired farm solved the problem. There are no signs on the gate indicating the nature of the place, for fear of vandalism by fanatic Christians who hold flash-mob services at the doors of Jurema temples, shouting through loudspeakers that works of the devil are performed there. The simple block house has a table at the back, to the right of the entrance, with the usual profusion of images, pipes, glasses, and goblets that juremeiros call princes and princesses, symbolizing the "cities" of Jurema, that is, mythical places inhabited by enchanted beings.

The guiding entity of the house is Mestre Carlos. The property already has a few jurema trees, both black and white, planted "from seed" by Dona Raquel. She lights a cigar and begins to walk, smoking, among the low-growing trees, watering them as she sings Jurema songs she learned from Rita do Acais when she moved to Alhandra in the 1980s, or that she receives from spirits when she is irradiated, that is, in the presence of an enchanted being. Twice a month, or whenever someone is in great need, she performs what she calls "louvação" (praise rituals) on the property. She does not engage in "left-hand" works, meaning she only works for good, never for harm: "A juremeiro is not like in Umbanda, it's more natural, pure science."

She planted the jurema trees from seeds brought from "cities"—the name given to consecrated trees—to preserve their descendants and to ensure, in the future, material for preparing wine or liqueur from the plant. The second beverage, milder, is the one she regularly uses in her rituals. The stronger one, made from the root, she reserves for treating "very obsessed people," when more energy is needed. The liqueur, which I tasted from a small bottle she gifted me on the eve of my departure from Alhandra, has the sweet vegetal flavor suggested by its name.

Dona Raquel says she manifested mediumship around the age of seven, without knowing what it was. An "Indian grandmother," who gathered roots in the forest to make her herbal remedies and syrups, considered it natural that the girl saw people adorned with feathers, dancing, whom no one else could see. It's Pena Branca, normal, the elderly relative would say. Word spread that the girl had a "good current" (mediumship), and people began to call her to pray when someone fell ill, and the sick would recover. "It was the entity that did that. It really started with the indigenous part, my ancestors," says Dona Raquel, "but it was only in Alhandra that I came to understand what the science of Jurema is."

It is not only on the Cantinho that Dona Raquel practices her science. On Wednesdays, she leads Jurema sessions at the Alhandra Spiritist Center, in the second part of a ceremony that begins with Kardecist prayers and lectures. The back of the hall, on the city's main avenue, is covered by a blue curtain and displays a sign with the word "Welcome." Rows of white plastic chairs line the side walls: to the right as you enter sit the mediums (three women and four men); to the left, the visitors, almost exclusively women, all barefoot. I sit apart, near the door, with only Nayanne Alves dos Santos beside me, the 29-year-old woman who introduced me to Dona Raquel.

Standing in the middle of the semicircle, the healer asserts that Jesus was the greatest juremeiro, the greatest medium and complains about those who say that those gathered there are not Christians. A man stands up and leads a Lord's Prayer, another reads psychographed letters from Bezerra de Menezes.[41,42] A boy of about five plays in the hall without anyone scolding him, crawling with a toy car in hand, lying on the floor, bothering his mother, a medium focused on the ceremony.

Dona Raquel speaks in defense of the healer's profession, in which there is no rest, with people knocking on her door at five in the morning in need of help. Jurema was supposed to be our religion, the religion of Brazil, she says. "Many people think that by destroying [Jurema] they end the sacred, but they don't, the science does not end. Allan Kardec studied and proved that there is life after death." She then begins to sing Jurema songs:

> *In the São Francisco River I dove*
> *I went to the bottom*
> *I went to fetch the black man from Angola*
> *The whole Nation came*
> *Jurema blossomed*
> *From Angico to Vajucá*
> *Unravel this chain*
> *Let the masters work*

Accompanied only by the sound of singing and clapping, in a ritual where no one drinks jurema wine, at least seven mediums begin to receive entities, all at the same time, including Nayanne, who incorporates her master and guide, Zé Bebim. She walks awkwardly through the hall, different from the exuberant style adopted by the other mediums. Dona Raquel comes to ask if I want to talk or ask him anything; I almost say no, nothing specific to consult, but I get up and go. Zé Bebim says he wishes me success in my work of dissemination and that I narrate with great wisdom everything I am witnessing.

During the session at the Spiritist Center, an impressive trance scene occurred: a young woman visiting for the first time began to leap and wave her arms in front of Dona Raquel, as if attacking her, and she restrained her movements. The episode escalated, and the celebrant asked for help from those present, both incorporated and not, who held the young woman and eventually made her to sit in a chair brought to the center of the hall. It took four to six people to restrain her at various times. I could only hear her anguished plea: "He wants to take me, he wants to take me. He is suffering. Don't let him!" They sprayed her with a large amount of perfumed liquid called lavender. The youngest medium repeatedly ran his hands over her arms and legs, while others did the same on her head. They spoke to the spirit, which Nayanne said was a fierce caboclo, without doctrine.

The anthropologist Estêvão Palitot, from the Federal University of Paraíba (UFPB), upon hearing the account, would later say in an interview that it is common in these rituals for a kind of reenactment of the colonial process to occur, in which more evolved beings of European culture—in this case, those of the Kardecist tradition—domesticate and impose doctrine on wild, untamed beings, who accept it in their own recalcitrant way. The young woman had two episodes during that session, between which she collapsed, prostrate, in her original visitor's chair.

After manifesting Zé Bebim and helping to restrain the fierce caboclo, Nayanne returned to sit beside me. Her goal, she says, is to be an independent medium, without affiliating herself with any house under the guidance of a padrinho or madrinha of Jurema. The young woman works with Dona Raquel to develop her mediumship, which she discovered in the usual way: she had visions as a child, which her mother identified as dead people, as well as frequent fainting spells and convulsions. She was later diagnosed with depression, anxiety, and panic disorder, and only recovered when she began to receive guidance after coming into contact with the Sacred Jurema at the age of 23 or 24—five years, therefore, before she recounted her life to me in an interview.

She met Dona Raquel and discovered another aspect, which she calls clean Jurema, clean Umbanda, an Afro-based religion, "real science," grounded and authentic. It's not a terreiro, she explains, it's under the jurema tree, the way like the Indians used to do, white garments, pipe, herbs, and cachaça. They hold ceremonies without drums, using only handclaps and the maracá. The young woman began her training with what she calls spiritual work: cleansings, herbal baths, and strengthening rituals.

A month and a half later, at the Cantinho dos Benzedores, she received her first entity, a master who made a commitment with her, and she with him, to work in healing, walking a steady path. It was Zé Bebim, who asked her for a head covering (hat) and a pipe, teaching her how to prepare it, although he prefers cigars. He likes cachaça and carries the bottle under his arm, but she assures that she does not feel drunk after disincorporating the master, even after taking several sips of the spirit. Although he is her guide, there is no exclusivity: Nayanne also receives gypsies, old black spirits, Mestra Menina, and two exus. "You need to know how to walk so you don't receive an entity that isn't from the right-hand line," she says. For this, she keeps her body clean through baths for energetic discharge, that is, to rid herself of the energy of the person she healed and not become ill herself.

The young woman divides her time between Alhandra, where her five-year-old daughter lives with her grandmother, and João Pessoa, where she carries out much of her activism in social movements. She has worked as a campaign aide and parliamentary advisor, call center operator, and Uber driver. Her main cause is to fight the disunity among terreiro peoples, not only among practitioners of the Sacred Jurema, who are always harassed by the aggressive intolerance of some neo-Pentecostals. There was a time when she couldn't even go out on the street without people shouting "There goes the macumbeira!" She helps find lawyers when terreiros are vandalized and complains about the lack of public support for religions under attack, with authorities claiming they practice evil. She achieved a major victory three months before the interview, when the Alhandra City Council approved Law 0678, establishing Jurema Day on September 22.

A Family Tragedy and the Preservation of Faith by Father Ciriaco

Almost everything is small and modest in the house of João José da Silva, in Alhandra. The city's oldest juremeiro master, known as Mestre Ciriaco, a short man with a face deeply lined by a life marked by tragedy, exudes vitality at 85 years. Dressed in white and barefoot, he introduces his wife Maria das Dores to the visitors arriving for the Jurema session, which would begin 45 min after the scheduled time, 7 p.m.; the enchanted beings apparently unconcerned with punctuality. Dorinha, as Ciriaco calls her, has the pale face of someone very ill, a disproportionately swollen belly, and speaks in a low, breathless voice, recounting a litany of doctor visits and inconclusive diagnoses.

The room where the ceremony will take place is no more than three by four meters. It is filled with half a dozen plastic chairs and ritual objects—simple painted plaster statuettes, bottles of cachaça and sparkling wine, ceramic bowls with pipes and maracás, candles—scattered on the floor. At the back, to the left, under the window facing the street, a long table displays the usual variety of symbols dear to Catimbó, or Sacred Jurema: glasses of water, pipes, a bell, figures of orixás and Catholic saints—Saint Lucy, Saint George, Saint Sebastian, Our Lady, Jesus Christ—bundles of candles, and white flowers in a vase atop the blue and white cloth. Ciriaco settles onto the stool at the right head of the table, which, unlike the opposite end, is not against the wall, and his feet barely touch the floor.

The jurema practitioner Dona Raquel, the main guest that Tuesday, December 6, 2022, is also dressed entirely in white. While waiting for the session to begin, she strikes up a conversation with Ciriaco, asking about the police repression he suffered before opening his former temple, the Centro Espírita Rei Malunguinho. Catimbozeiros were hunted like drug traffickers are today, the master recounts. On the plantation where he grew up in Itambé (state of Pernambuco), the land owner wanted nothing to do with macumba and would order it stopped, refusing to allow it. "But I'm going to do it, because God wants it," Ciriaco would reply. Things only improved after 1966—by then he was living in Alhandra—when a Religious Freedom Law was enacted, regulating the practice in the state of Paraíba and requiring registration with the Federation of Afro-Brazilian Cults. He recalls that at one point there were 86 mediums in the temple, his spiritual godchildren.

More guests arrive and the ritual begins. "Thanks to God, our Lord Jesus Christ. May everything be protected by our Lord Jesus Christ and the powers of the Sacred Jurema," proclaims Ciriaco. "Who is greater than God?" he asks. "No one," the attendees reply. At no point is any beverage, with or without black jurema, consumed. Still seated, the master's hands begin to tremble over the table, the movement intensifying until the shaking echoes as slaps on the tabletop, at which point the medium whistles and leaps to his feet. An assistant supports him from behind and moves the stool away to give him space. With the entity incorporated—one of several that will visit Ciriaco's "matter" (body)—he staggers in the limited space, speaks in an altered voice, and addresses Dona Raquel, as if inviting her to receive her guides as well, but she maintains the posture of a mere observer, as she explains to the master manifested by the host. He agrees and blesses the visitor.

Returning to the bench, the drumming of hands on the table and the whistle are repeated during the disincorporation. The scenes unfold with other masters and caboclos of Jurema and blessings for those present in the room. The so-called cleansing of bodies is performed by Ciriaco taking the visitor's hands and spinning three times with his partner, without letting go of hands, passing their forearms over their heads. At a certain point, Zé Pelintra appears, Dona Raquel explains to me. I am summoned by the master to stand and give him my hands. I comply, agreeing with his words of welcome and thanking him for his wishes for good work in Alhandra, nodding my head. As I am about to return to my seat, the entity challenges me: "You don't believe it's really me, do you?" The answer comes spontaneously: "Who am I not to believe, Seu Zé?".

Amid many Jurema songs and Christian prayers, the only person besides Ciriaco to incorporate is Dorinha, in an astonishing transformation. The woman, previously confined to her chair, throws herself to the floor, where she begins to laugh and harangue with a powerful voice against evils and doctors, her legs bent backward at an improbable angle. She asks for a small wooden pestle, which she strikes forcefully on the floor to emphasize her complaints and imprecations. It is the most striking scene of the night, and I am so taken aback by the metamorphosis that I forget to record it on video. Where does all that energy come from, covering the patient's temples with sweat as she is momentarily eclipsed? It is Pilão Deitado, they explain later, an enchanted master at the death of the cangaceiro (bandit) of the same nickname, who in life is said to have roamed the backlands with Captain Antônio Silvino more than a century ago.

While he maintained his temple dedicated to Malunguinho, Ciriaco held ceremonies every fifteen days, alternating between Jurema and "for the saint," in deference to Dorinha's deep involvement with orixás, exus, and pombajiras. The juremeiro told anthropologist Sandro Guimarães de Salles, for his doctoral research in 2010[43]:

I only sing for Exu at the opening of the Jurema because Dorinha is [of] orixá, you know... [In] Jurema there's no place for Exu... but because of her, who works with Pombajira, and all that, right? But I don't like it, I'm not a fanatic. Now, caboclo and master, that's my path, right? I'll go with it to the end of my life.

That's not quite how life turned out, says the man, now bitter, in our conversation for this book, thirteen years after the interview with Salles, as he recounts why he had closed his temple a year earlier, in 2021, and now only performed domestic table sessions, revisiting the times when catimbozeiros carried out their rites hidden inside their homes.

"They killed my son, who was a great juremeiro," he says, "they killed my daughter-in-law." João José da Silva Filho, Pai Jonas Ciriaco, was shot dead along with his wife in front of their house, murders that remained unsolved. The father refuses to give further details about the deaths, but rumors in the town suggest connections with disputes involving local politicians of Evangelical faith. When directly asked about religious persecution, Ciriaco evades the question, bitterness written on his face: "Great person, I can't say anything about that. I can't accuse anyone. If I were sure, I would explain, but I don't know." His masters, the caboclos, the orixás, did not warn him, he says, disheartened. "My beloved son, who studied so much. He knew how to do everything, a great juremeiro, I was the one who trained him. I had more than a hundred filhos de santo. He played the drum, he was my ogã."

In Afro-Brazilian religions, ogãs are assistants in the rituals responsible for drumming and singing. The son helped his father in the terreiro, but then he started to faint, says Mestre Ciriaco, referring to episodes of fainting and absences usually interpreted as signs of mediumship. "I said, 'my son, you are a medium and your saint is Ogum.'".

Thus, the story of the owner of the terreiro repeated itself, who would fall into trance in the fields when he still worked at the sugarcane mill in Itambé. Taken to the Pernambuco juremeiro master Zé Pedro, he recounts that the master told his family that the young man's illness was a spiritual current. He began working in Jurema, assisting Zé Pedro, and after moving to Alhandra, he helped Dona Zefinha de Tiíno, also known as Mestra Jardecilha, from a famous terreiro in the city, where his grandson Lucas still works. Zé Pedro sent him to fetch black jurema in the Muriçoca forest, a place Ciriaco did not even know. Guided by a master, Ciriaco found the "city" of black jurema. He asked permission, took the bark, extracted the root, and prepared the wine himself as the entity had taught him.

I ask if the recipe is secret and he replies that it is not, but that he only works on the right side (not on the left, meaning magic to do harm): "Take the bark and put it in a container with water, or another ingredient—some people add cachaça. It's good to have a little jurema," he explains with a broad smile, raising his thumb to his mouth in the universal gesture for drinking. "Add more sugarcane molasses, add fennel, add cloves, add sweet sugarcane juice, add whatever you want." He recommends waiting three days after preparation. Then you can also add water and wait seven days for it to mature.

Ciriaco says he only drinks jurema during the ritual, but that he does not need it, no sir, to channel a spirit. In fact, during the table work witnessed at his home, the drink was not available. "A medium is already made. We're playing here and we go fetch him as if we were going from here to Dona Raquel's house [far away]," he explains. On his refusal to work with the left:

"I promised Jesus Christ I would not do harm. For any illness, the fellow [himself] is there to provide [healing]." At my request, he sings two Jurema songs, the first of which was received by Ciriaco himself:

Jurema has, Jurema gives
A good caboclo to work
Come down, caboclo, come down in the juremá
The caboclo is good to work
I was in the middle of the forest
In the middle of the vines
Oh mother, rock me
For I want to be rocked
Rock me, mother, rock me
For I want to be rocked

Ciriaco was thirty or forty years old, he does not remember exactly, when he opened his own Centro Espírita Rei Malunguinho. He paid the Umbanda Federation, from which he says he still has the receipts. Once, he was questioned by the police chief, a skeptic, about his healings, and he replied by asking them to bring any sick person: "If they don't get better, you can arrest me. Back when there was no license, Hail Maria, the authorities would come after you." He says he personally knew famous masters of Alhandra, such as Zé Francisco, Cavalão, Cabeça Branca, and Rita do Acais, to whom he claims to have taught how to conduct the gira. "I met Maria do Acais, the Indian. Very beautiful person, beautiful master. I went to Flósculo, to Zezinho do Acais."

Evangelical Attacks and Rivalry Between Jurema Temples in Alhandra

Seen from Manuel Guedes Street, the house where the Templo Espírita de Jurema Mestra Jardecilha is located looks like an ordinary residence, and, in fact, in the front part of the property, Severina Paulino de Souza, known as Nina, the daughter of the renowned master, lives there. An external corridor on the left side leads to a large backyard, with two separate buildings and several jurema trees established as "cities" (consecrated jurema trees) dedicated to Mestra Jardecilha herself and to Maria do Acais, but also to the masters Major do Dias, Manuel Cadete, José da Paz, Zezinho do Acais, Zé Pelintra, Cesário, Canito, Zé Quati, Bom Florar, Felipiano, and Malunguinho, according to the description by Francisco Sales de Lima Segundo.[44]

With the demolition of the buildings on the Acais farm and the clearing of the "cities" near the PB-034 highway, the Temple, located within the urban perimeter of Alhandra, came to concentrate the largest number of consecrated jurema trees in the region.

At the back, to the right, there is a chapel dedicated to Our Lady of the Immaculate Conception. To the left, behind the cross bearing the inscription "God Save the Cross of the Lords Masters of the Sacred Jurema of this Temple" and the House of Souls and Old Blacks (a small, closed cubicle for offerings, just over a meter high), is the hall used for the Torés de Caboclo, as Nina refers to the gatherings, a festivity featuring the playing of ilus drums where Tapuias, Canindés, and the masters play, deliver messages and teachings, and drink their jurema, as the mistress of the house recounts.

To the right of those entering the hall, which has a white ceramic floor, are two Jurema tables, the oldest of which belonged to Mestra Jardecilha herself. Nina says that the piece of furniture, covered with a white cloth and holding glasses of water, gourds, pipes, candles, small ceramic cups, and painted plaster statuettes representing Zé Pelintra, Saint George, old black spirits, and a cabocla, is made of hardwood and is over 150 years old: "Everything here has meaning. There are no crystal glasses on her table, it is humble. It was not meant to show off. Jurema is charity. If you raise your nose, it's easier to fall, you can't see the ground." In her view, spirits do not need flashy clothes, as in some African-derived religions; what is needed is prayer, is song. "Everything here is my mother, [she] could be enchanted in any of these trees."

Jardecilha Luíza de Sousa was born on June 11, 1934, and died on August 27, 1988. Also known as Dona Zefa de Tiíno, Dona Zefinha, Madrinha Zefinha, or Tia Zefa, she began to manifest mediumistic abilities as a child, a story of encounters with spirits that is repeated in the biographies of nearly every juremeiro who incorporates entities. In her case, her guide was Manuel Cadete, but Nina says her mother also received exus and pombajiras. She was known for her simplicity; between 1965 and 1986, she held torés in her kitchen, where she also welcomed poor people, offering them consultations and food.

She was a friend of Friar Anastácio, who in the 1970s and 1980s was responsible for the parish of Our Lady of the Assumption and a leading figure in the progressive group of bishop Dom Helder Câmara. She constantly brought children to be baptized by the friar, becoming godmother to more than six hundred of them. She even maintained good relations with the evangelicals of that time, when it was not a problem for Pastor Sebastião or the Catholic priest to visit her home. She only opened the José da Paz Umbanda

Temple in the 1980s, according to Lima Segundo, the same period in which she became an inspector for the Federation of Afro-Brazilian Cults of Paraíba, a clear demonstration that Jurema and Umbanda not only coexist but are intertwined in the mysticism of the Northeast.

Her daughter Nina was sixty years old when she gave the interview for this book, walking through the yard and pointing out each significant spot, not without first asking to take a bath and put on a clean white dress for the video recording. She takes care of everything there, especially the herb garden she uses for ritual baths, which, according to her, must be planted and harvested at the right time and moon phase. But she says she is tired after 34 years of struggle to preserve the place under continuous attack from religious intolerance. Everyone wants to tear it down, she laments. "You give up everything, your leisure, sleeping a little longer."

Nine cameras were installed to monitor the property, but she says people would cut the wires, throw bombs, and threaten to kill her children. She reluctantly reveals that many of the problems with neopentecostalists come from neighboring relatives who, like her, inherited a share of the land acquired by their great-great-grandparents, but without a satisfactory agreement. A wall was built over the root of a jurema tree; another "city" was destroyed. In 2011, she paid four thousand reais for four square meters, money partly raised from donors, in an attempt to resolve one of the disputes. She went to Brasília seeking support, took part in protests, asked the police for help, all to no avail. "Will a police officer want to protect a catimbozeiro?".

Today's police neglect still echoes the past of state persecution that followed the relentless cultural repression exercised by the Catholic Church over four centuries—unsuccessfully, as evidenced by the survival of indigenous and African religious practices. In 1938, a year after the death of Maria do Acais, when Jurema was still called Catimbó in Alhandra and Xangô in Recife, the head of the São Paulo Folklore Research Mission, Luiz Saia, collected in just one month from local newspapers eight reports of raids and arrests[45]:

- "Several Xangôs closed by the police" (*Diário de Pernambuco*, Feb. 13);
- "Catimbó, Xangô, and the stomping of Macumba" (*Diário da Manhã*, Feb. 15);
- "City Chronicle: Police Continue Campaign to Suppress Low Magic" (*Jornal do Comércio*, Feb. 20);
- "Police Investigations into the Closure of Xangô and Catimbó Houses" (*Diário da Manhã*, Feb. 22);

- "Two Catimbó Centers Closed on Avenida Norte: Large Amount of Ritual Material, Herbs, and Consultation Cards Seized" (*Diário de Pernambuco*, Feb. 22);
- "Cleansing Our Customs: Police Raid Two Catimbó Centers" (*Jornal do Comércio*, Feb. 22);
- "Against the Practice of Low Spiritism: Police Raid the Kings' Magi Center of the Well-Known Catimbó Practitioner Caetana" (*Diário de Pernambuco*, Mar. 8);
- "Relentless Crackdown on Exploiters of Popular Belief: Police Continue Operations Against Low Spiritism Centers. A Well-Known Catimbó Practitioner Detained" (*Jornal do Comércio*, Mar. 19).

The term "catimbó" is regarded as bad, sorcery, magic, propagation of evil, something dark, laments José Lucas Paulino de Souza, son of Nina, who continues to venerate the masters of his grandmother Jardecilha. At 27 years old at the time of the interview, he is also a Candomblé priest, but does not practice Candomblé at the terreiro in Alhandra, only at the terreiro he attends in the city of Goiana (Pernambuco), 28 kilometers away. "I don't even mix the liturgical environment. 'Amen,' not 'axé.' I don't use anything from Candomblé here in the terreiro. Ilu, not atabaque." He says he knows well what religious intolerance is: "We have to worship during the day so as not to disturb the neighbors. We will never be understood or defended. Evangelicals park cars [in front of the house] for flash mobs, with loudspeakers. I have already been threatened with death."

Flash mob services are improvised ceremonies performed by evangelicals in Alhandra as an opportunity for many conversions. They take place daily on the city's streets, each day in a different location, featuring preaching of the Gospel, singing, and testimonies, inviting residents to convert to the evangelical faith, as several believers reported to Luiz Francisco da Silva Junior.[46] According to this author's survey in 2010, there were ten Catholic churches, twenty evangelical churches, and nine Jurema/Umbanda centers in the urban and rural areas of Alhandra.

Nina's son and Jardecilha's grandson reject the title of Pai Lucas, preferring to be called Lucas Juremeiro. He makes crafts related to the cult, such as pipes carved from the hard wood of the jurema tree, which he sells online (his Instagram account had over 2,900 followers as of September 2023). He is concerned about the loss of Jurema's identity due to the growing influence of Umbanda, which he traces to the 1970s, and currently with the neo-shamanic or recreational trend that uses jurema as a drug, whether in the form of black jurema and Syrian rue teas or as crystals extracted from the former for smoking in pipes, usually glass, known as "changa." There are YouTube videos teaching how to make jurema wine with Syrian rue, which completely departs from the indigenous liturgy meant for contacting ancestors, not for recreation, he complains. "They take the cultural context, squeeze it, squeeze it, and reduce it to a tea that gets you high, an external trance, an ecstasy." He says, however, that the syncretism that led to the emergence of the spiritist tables, when Jurema ceased to be practiced in the forest and on the ground, was a justified survival strategy in the face of police persecution. When Spiritism arrived in Brazil in the nineteenth century, it was well received because it was European, he argues. The police had no issue with table sessions, so Jurema practitioners began to work indoors—means by which Jurema reinvented itself and survived. Instead of the maracá, the bell, the handbell, or glasses of water. When the police arrived, there was no physical evidence of witchcraft. Many Jurema practitioners died at the time because they confronted the authorities. Flósculo and Zezinho were regarded as pagan witches, he laments. Lucas attributes to "the wisdom of Black people" the use of tronqueiras (pieces of tree trunks common among terreiro sacred objects), when it became impossible to venerate living jurema trees because the police would cut them down. In the quilombos, he says, the two traditions merged, and Africans passed on to Indigenous people the practice of sacrifices—which did not exist in Catimbó—to give life to a piece of cut wood, to enchant it. Today, it is religious intolerance led by neo-Pentecostals that threatens this encounter of religiosities from three continents amalgamated in Catimbó/Jurema:

> They want to remove the Christian tradition from Jurema, believing it does not belong. Even knowing that the Indigenous peoples were forcibly catechized, we must understand that the Christian element in Jurema was mixed, completely transformed, and intensified by our ancestors.

Eriberto Carvalho Ribeiro, known as Pai Beto de Xangô, had scheduled the interview in the Cidade Verde II neighborhood, in João Pessoa (Paraíba), for 3:30 p.m. and suggested I arrive a little earlier. I knocked at 3 p.m. on the house, which has a statue of Christ on the street, next to a wall covered in light brown tiles, topped by the canopy of a large black jurema tree planted inside, but no one answered. I asked for help from the young man at the neighboring barbershop, who said he was probably sleeping. Soon, a group of five people dressed in white arrived, carrying what seemed to be containers of food. I entered with them, and one of the young men began to show me the spacious rooms on the ground floor that house the minimalist collection of the Paraíba Museum of Afro-Brazilian and Indigenous Culture (MUPAI).

Among the modest collection is the bell from the Acais chapel, a source of great resentment for some juremeiros from Alhandra toward Pai Beto, who calls himself Guardian of the Sacred Jurema and brought the relics from the Jurema mecca to his house-museum in the capital of Paraíba.

Pai Beto appeared, descending the staircase that leads to his quarters, and we entered the library lined with blue tiles, with a table adorned with green, yellow, and white beaded necklaces, where the priest sat in a high-backed iron chair topped with a small double-bladed axe (symbol of orixá Xangô). Tall and strong at 49, he wore white shorts and shirt, as well as a lace cap. On his left bicep, an armband with cowrie shells. In contrast to other Jurema worship sites I visited in Northeastern Brazil, this one impresses with what could be called opulence. Pai Beto maintains two other sites in Alhandra: the Temple of the Twelve Kingdoms of the Holy and Sacred Jurema, with its four columns on a white façade separated from Claudionor Falsar Street by an ornate iron fence and gate, and the Reino do Bom Florar site, where he erected what he claims to be the largest master cross in the world.

His initiation into the orixá cult is recent, just over a decade. Before that, he worked only with Jurema, into which he was initiated by Maria dos Prazeres Santos Soares, known as Mãe Maria do Peixe. He says he began visiting Alhandra, traveling the 41 km from the Paraíba capital, because the town is the birthplace of the Sacred Jurema, but he became concerned about the precarious state of holy sites such as the chapel and the Acais farm and the Zezinho do Acais memorial. "Cities" (jurema trees) were being cut down, and there were reports of attacks motivated by religious intolerance from the evangelical segment of the population, such as members of the Assembleia de Deus[47] who began settling in the region in the 1950s.[48] Pai Beto was one of the organizers, on June 20, 2009, of the Peace March in defense of one of the jurema trees in Mestra Jardecilha's terreiro, threatened with being cut down during the division of land among heirs who had converted to the evangelical faith. That same year, with the listing of the site and chapel of Maria do Acais as heritage, he was one of the leaders of the Victory March—a Pyrrhic victory, it must be said, because the house of the pioneering priestess had already been demolished.

Pai Beto says he decided to build the Temple of the Twelve Kingdoms of the Holy and Sacred Jurema in Alhandra, with its "sumptuous" façade, as he describes it, to make it clear that being a juremeiro or catimbozeiro was not something only for the poor, for those who have nothing in life: "I wanted to show the evangelicals that it's not like that," he says. "When someone passes in front of [an evangelical church], they know it's a religious temple." There, he holds rituals every two weeks. Followers from João Pessoa travel to the site by car, which prompts comments in the town, even from some juremeiros, saying that at the Temple of the Twelve Kingdoms, only those with a car can enter. "My fight is against religious intolerance, to reclaim Jurema. I don't get involved in anyone's gossip; I've been in Alhandra for eighteen years."

He only uses jurema wine on special occasions, such as initiation baptisms and other internal works of the terreiro, or to give spiritual passes to invited people suffering from depression, obsession, or persistent headaches, to awaken the person to life. But only in small quantities, purely symbolically. Like his rival Lucas, he criticizes those who use jurema as a psychedelic tea, adding, for example, Syrian rue, or who abuse alcohol in Jurema ceremonies: "The one who has the right to drink whiskey is a Guardian of the Street [Exu]. The one who has the right to drink a glass of champagne—I'm talking about a glass, not a bottle—is pombajira, is Maria Padilha," he asserts. "The one who has the right to drink jurema wine is the caboclo, is the one in need. If someone feels unwell, you can't convince me that [the use] is sacred. It's a drug. They are opportunistic juremeiros."

At the end of the interview, on December 8, 2022, the day of Our Lady of the Conception (Iemanjá, in Afro-Brazilian syncretism), he sings the requested two Jurema songs of his choice, the first of which is usually sung on the beach of Tambaba during the initiation of juremeiros:

> *At the bottom of the sea there is a stone*
> *Beneath the stone lies knowledge*
> *Whoever is troubled in this world*
> *Ask God to enter into science*
> *Sustain me, Jurema, sustain me*
> *Hold me, Juremá, hold me*
> *The church of Acais only opens from behind*
> *And the patroness of the church is Maria do Acais*
> *Maria do Acais, through her I can call*
> *She never deceived anyone, so as not to deceive anyone*
> *So I keep running, I can't take it anymore*
> *I will take my despair to Maria do Acais*

Three months after the interview at MUPAI, Pai Beto allows me to accompany him during a Sacred Jurema ritual at the Casa do Catimbó terreiro in the remote neighborhood of Mangabeira 2, in João Pessoa. The hall is very bright, measuring between 150 and 200 square meters, with a shiny white ceramic floor. One of the walls displays a poster listing the rules to be followed by the sons and daughters of the terreiro, which also bears the name Ylé Asé Sangò Ògòdò (Ilê Axé Xangô Ogodô). Among these, rule number six stands out: "It is strictly forbidden to talk about other people's lives." Along two walls, there are rows of about fifty white plastic chairs; in the center of the hall, a smaller circle with fourteen of them and a kind of iron armchair that appears identical to the one Pai Beto sat in for the interview the previous December. At the back, a shelf shaped like a six-pointed star (the Seal of Solomon) holds multicolored images of saints, masters, caboclos, and old black spirits. The floor in the middle of the smaller circle of chairs is covered with green leaves, statuettes, and straw hats.

Between 6:30 and 7:00 p.m., the hall fills up, with more than thirty people present. The initiates settle in the inner circle, men in light trousers and floral shirts, women in white skirts or dresses, some with turbans and patterned blouses. There is a certain buzz when Pai Beto arrives, snapping his fingers three times in front of a door covered with the image of Xangô and lighting candles on the shelf behind his metal throne. He opens the ceremony with a welcome and a speech that reinforces the sixth rule of conduct on the wall: "Life is made of choices. Each person is responsible for their actions. The cursed tongue: after everything is said, there is no point in trying to blame life, God, or your family for your mistakes," he preaches. "Take responsibility for your actions. Having faith and exercising self-control is all that remains. There is a lot of energy in life just to be, simply. When you die, it's over."

He follows with greeting songs to Exu to open the Jurema ritual, accompanied only by clapping (two drums in the background remain covered with white cloths):

> *At the gate I left my sentinel*
> *But I left Tranca-Rua*
> *Watching over the gate*
> *I was standing at the crossroads*
> *A rooster came and pecked my foot*
> *You play with Exu because you want to*
> *Exu is a man, not a woman*

The songs and clapping continue until 7:40 p.m., when Pai Beto exclaims: "Exu wants, Exu can, Exu commands." A woman in the inner circle bursts out laughing and begins to shake her shoulders, lifting one side more than the other, initiating a series of spirit incorporations, in this case a pombajira. A young man in pink trousers adopts similar gestures and walks around the hall, after a woman in a yellow blouse, possibly an assistant to Pai Beto, provides him with a kind of white tunic or dress over his regular clothes. "To mess with Maria Padilha is to mess with the lid of your [own] coffin," proclaims Beto de Xangô. The woman in yellow whispers something in the young man's ear, who then disengages from the spirit. The master of ceremonies intones:

Open the gate, Exu is leaving
Exu has drunk, Exu has eaten, Exu is leaving

It is already 8:20 p.m. when Jurema's work proper begins. The assistant moves around the hall offering scented water to each of those present. Pai Beto lights a pipe and, blowing into the bowl, spreads the smoke that pours out through the mouthpiece, turning 360° around himself. One of the young men in the inner circle begins to sing the Jurema points. The incorporations resume, and now it is the turn of the masters, such as Zé Bebim. By 9:30 p.m., at least five people are "irradiated," walking around the hall. Two more women from the audience receive entities, to whom the assistant in yellow attends, wearing the same white robe and a hat. At 9:50 p.m., the hats of the seven mediums begin to be collected, and Pai Beto announces that Jurema is leaving, singing a variation of an Umbanda point:

I close my work
With God and Our Lady
I close my work
With God and the Blacks of Angola

At exactly 10:00 p.m., the ceremony ends, leaving a certain sense of astonishment in the air at the punctuality and the obedience of the entities to Pai Beto's commands, in contrast to the somewhat chaotic session at Mestre Ciriaco's house in Alhandra. Sales open at the entrance table, and I buy a traditional pipe for twenty reais. At no point was there any consumption of a beverage prepared with black jurema, a clear indication that the wine shared with the ancestors is now sublimated into a cloud of symbols and echoes of the religiosity that survived among the Indigenous peoples of the Northeast and was strengthened through alliance with the enslaved people brought from Africa.

Notes

1. Rodrigo Grünewald, *Jurema.* Campinas: Mercado de Letras, 2020. p. 185.
2. Luís da Câmara Cascudo, *Meleagro: Pesquisa do Catimbó e notas da magia branca no Brasil.* Rio de Janeiro: Agir, 1978. p. 37.
3. Mário de Andrade, *Música de Feitiçaria no Brasil.* São Paulo: Livraria Martins Editora, 1963. p. 33.

4. José Ribeiro, *Catimbó, Magia do Nordeste*. Rio de Janeiro: Pallas, 1991. pp. 26–7.

5. Mário de Andrade, *O Turista Aprendiz*. Belo Horizonte: Garnier, 2021. p. 194.

6. Luís da Câmara Cascudo, *Meleagro: Pesquisa do Catimbó e notas da magia branca no Brasill*, pp. 51 and 55.

7. José Ribeiro, *Catimbó,, Magia do Nordeste*, p. 28.

8. Mário de Andrade, *O Turista Aprendiz*, pp. 195–8.

9. Idem, *Música de Feitiçaria no Brasil*, pp. 34–5.

10. Ibid., pp. 58–9.

11. Álvaro Carlini, *Cachimbo Maracá: O Catimbó da Missão (1938)*. São Paulo: CCSP, 1993. p. 72.

12. Sandro Guimarães de Salles, *ÀSombra da Jurema Encantada: Mestres juremeiros na Umbanda de AlhandraÀ*. Recife: Editora UFPE, 2010. p. 125.

13. Ibid.

14. Luiz Antonio Simas, *Umbandas: Uma História do Brasil*. Rio de Janeiro: Civilização Brasileira, 2023. pp. 76–7.

15. Ibid., pp. 77–8.

16. Reginaldo Prandi, *Brasil Africano: Deuses, sacerdotes, seguidores*. Itanhaém, SP: Arché, 2022. p. 102.

17. Ibid., p. 110.

18. Pai Rodney, "Maria Padilha: ela é bonita, ela é mulher". *Carta Capital*, Mar. 30, 2018. Available at: https://www.cartacapital.com.br/blogs/dialogos-da-fe/maria-padilha-ela-e-bonita-ela-e-mulher/. Accessed: Dec. 20, 2024.

19. Sandro Guimarães de Salles, *À Sombra da Jurema Encantada*, p. 122.

20. Ibid., p. 123.

21. Clélia Moreira Pinto, "A Jurema Sagrada". In: Clarice Novaes da Mota, Ulysses Paulino de Albuquerque (Eds.), *As Muitas Faces da Jurema: Da espécie botânica à divindade afro-indígena*. Recife: Bagaço, 2002. p. 132.

22. Luiz Assunção, *O Reino dos Mestres: A tradição da Jurema na Umbanda nordestina*. Rio de Janeiro: Pallas, 2010. p. 231.

23. Francelino de Shapanan, "Entre caboclos e encantados: Mudanças recentes em cultos de caboclos na perspectiva de um chefe de terreiro.". In: Reginaldo Prandi (Ed.), *Encantaria Brasileira: O livro dos mestres, caboclos e encantados*. Rio de Janeiro: Pallas, 2011. p. 325.

24. Luiz Antonio Simas and Luiz Rufino, *Fogo no Mato: A ciência encantada das macumbas*. Rio de Janeiro: Mórula, 2018. p. 81.

25. Sandro Guimarães de Salles, *À Sombra da Jurema Encantada*, p. 122.

26. Alexandre L'Omi L'Odó, *Juremologia: Uma busca etnográfica para sistematização de princípios da cosmovisão da Jurema Sagrada*. Recife: Universidade Católica de Pernambuco, 2017. Master's thesis (Social Sciences). p. 206.

27. Sandro Guimarães de Salles, *À Sombra da Jurema Encantada*, p. 128.

28. Song collected by the Folklore Mission organized by Mário de Andrade and recorded by Álvaro Carlini in *Cachimbo e Maracá: O Catimbó da Missão (1938)*. São Paulo: CCSP, 1993. p. 173.

29. Alexandre L'Omi L'Odó, *Malunguinho: Pressupostos juremológicos para sua compreensão da Jurema Sagrada*. Olinda: Casa das Matas do Reis Malunguinho e Quilombo Cultural Malunguinho, 2022. pp. 43–7.

30. Sandro Guimarães de Salles, *À Sombra da Jurema Encantada*, p. 129.

31. Luís da Câmara Cascudo, *Meleagro: Pesquisa do Catimbó e notas da magia branca no Brasil*, p. 54.

32. Mário de Andrade, *Música de Feitiçaria no Brasil*, p. 119.

33. Luiz Assunção, *O Reino dos Mestres: A tradição da Jurema na Umbanda nordestina*. Rio de Janeiro: Pallas, 2010. p. 90.

34. Sandro Guimarães de Salles, *À Sombra da Jurema Encantada*, p. 116.

35. It is more common to find references to nutgrass (*Cyperus esculentus*) in the list of important plants for the Sacred Jurema.

36. Probably *Salzmannia nitida*.

37. Alexandre L'Omi L'Odó, *Juremologia*, pp. 186–7.

38. Rodrigo Grünewald, *Jurema*, p. 150.

39. Sandro Guimarães de Salles, *À Sombra da Jurema Encantadarema*, pp. 57–8.

40. Ibid., p. 211.

41. Adolfo Bezerra de Menezes Cavalcanti (1831–1900) was a physician and politician born in Ceará who built his career in Rio de Janeiro and presided over the Brazilian Spiritist Federation, founded in 1884.

42. Brazilian Spiritist Federation, *Adolfo Bezerra de Menezes: Apontamentos Biobibliográficos*. Available at: https://www.febnet.org.br/wp-content/uploads/2012/06/Adolfo-Bezerra-de-Menezes.pdf. Accessed: Dec. 20, 2024.

43. Sandro Guimarães de Salles, *Religião, espaço e transitividade: Jurema na Mata Norte de PE e Litoral Sul de PB*. Recife: UFPE, 2010. Doctoral thesis. p. 138.

44. Francisco Sales de Lima Segundo, *Memória e Tradição na Ciência da Jurema em Alhandra (PB): A cidade da Mestra Jardecilha*. João Pessoa: UFPB, 2015. Master's thesis (Anthropology). p. 152.

45. Álvaro Carlini, *Cachimbo e Maracá: O Catimbó da Missão (1938)*. São Paulo: CCSP, 1993. pp. 63–4, n. 2.

46. Luiz Francisco da Silva Junior,*A Jurema, o Culto e a Missa: Disputas pela identidade religiosa em Alhandra-PB (1980–2010)*. Campina Grande: UFCG, 2011. Master's thesis (History). p. 77.

47. According to the 2010 Census, evangelicals make up 21% of the population of Alhandra, which matches the national average in Brazil, but is above the rate for Paraíba, at 15%.

48. Ibid., p. 73.

The Power of Jurema in Indigenous Resistance in the Northeast

Intrigued by the cultural roots of the use of black jurema in the northeastern backlands, I made many trips to the region to learn about the centuries-old, or even millennia-old, Indigenous practices that still survive there and, more than that, thrive as a means of ethnic affirmation. One of my first excursions took me to the Academic Center of the Agreste (CAA, as in the Portuguese acronym, a campus of the Federal University of Pernambuco (UFPE) in Caruaru. Classes in the intercultural Indigenous teaching degree at the center are always preceded by a toré, a circular dance typical of the indigenous peoples of the Northeast. Students from various Indigenous groups usually sing and stomp their feet in the courtyard of the anthropology department, but on that Wednesday in November 2022, rain confined the toré to Sandro Guimarães de Salles's classroom. The Indigenous trainee teachers sang standing in place, without dancing, only playing the maracás, a musical instrument made from gourds and seeds, a large rattle that is another omnipresent element among the region's native peoples. One of the young men leads the point, or line, as the call-and-response songs between soloist and chorus are known in certain Afro-Indigenous rituals, in this case a question answered by the chorus of women:

Oh my beautiful caboclo
What are you doing here
I am wandering in foreign lands
Searching for my village

M. Leite, *The Psychedelic Science of the Jurema Tree*, Copernicus Books,
https://doi.org/10.1007/978-3-032-22705-8_3

The points follow one after another, sometimes initiated by a young woman:

> *Let us go with God and the Virgin Mary*
> *Let us go with God and Our Lady of Guidance*
> *Reina reiá, reina reina reiô*
> *Reina reiá, reina reina reiô*

The verses evoke mermaids, Cabocla Jurema, Saint George, Solomon, Mother of God, Our Lady of the Conception… At the end of each point, the maracás keep rattling as invocations are made: "Praised be Our Lord Jesus Christ/May He be praised forever." There are cheers for the pajés (shamans) and indigenous leaders. Someone shouts: "Hail the Orixás!", in reverence of deities from African origins.

The intercultural teaching degree began in 2009 and has already graduated two classes of Indigenous teachers from the twelve peoples present in Pernambuco. The academic calendar is governed by what is called pedagogical alternation between village and campus: in the last week of each month, students come to the CAA/UFPE for classes in the morning and afternoon, and in the other three weeks they work in their original villages. This back and forth serves two purposes: not to distance future graduates from Indigenous knowledge and practices, and to introduce them to the university and the city, in the hope that this will help reduce prejudice toward them in the general population.

João Batista do Nascimento, a Pankará from Lagoa village, travels about four hundred kilometers for his teaching degree classes, from the municipality of Carnaubeira da Penha to Caruaru. There are about 3,000 inhabitants in some fifty villages in the Pankará Indigenous Land of Serra do Arapuá, whose 15,000 hectares were identified in 2018 but still await official declaration and ratification.[1] At 48, though he appears younger, he seems to exert clear authority among his classmates. Son of the octogenarian shaman Manuelzinho do Cacheado (Manuel Antônio do Nascimento), he himself is now being initiated into the mysteries of jurema to also become a shaman: "Jurema is the foundation of our existence, the strength of our ancestry," he says in an interview during a class break. "Jurema is for everyone, but not everyone is for jurema," he adds, enigmatically. He confirms that the drink consumed by shamans during the torés is made from the root bark, but gives no further details, resorting to the secrecy with which these peoples almost always surround what they call the science of jurema. An important item in the rituals is the pipe, used to "cross" the jurema (blowing smoke in the shape of a cross over the vessel containing the drink), which also allows them to make contact with the ancestors. Incorporation of entities occurs in the rituals of his village, but only among those prepared to receive the enchanted beings.

Black jurema was once called *Mimosa hostilis*, perhaps because it defends itself with many thorns, and later its scientific name was softened to *Mimosa tenuiflora* (in allusion to the small flowers). Although both contain DMT, the so-called jurema wine, or ajucá, is different from the Amazon brew ayahuasca, or daime. From what little is known about traditional preparation methods, Indigenous peoples of the semi-arid Northeast prepare the wine cold, not by boiling, as is the case with the Amazonian tea. They squeeze the root bark in water at room temperature, which turns red and can even foam, according to some descriptions from those who have witnessed the process, about which shamans are reluctant to speak. It remains a mystery what the source of the enzyme inhibitor that degrades DMT in the original wine might have been. Two decades ago, a compound was found in jurema-preta itself, named yuremamine,[2] which could act as a MAO inhibitor, but this remains little more than a hypothesis regarding a little-studied plant and beverage. Other accounts suggest that wild cashew and passion fruit species, supposedly used by Indigenous peoples, may have served as psychedelic catalysts for DMT, but their ancient recipes are unknown.

"There is no Indigenous people in the Northeast who do not have this relationship with black jurema and the encantados, entities closely linked to Indigenous Jurema," explains Professor Salles in an interview during a class break. It reaffirms Indigenous value and identity, just like the toré. The languages, which in other parts of Brazil became the vehicle for maintaining "Indianness," eventually became extinct among Northeastern peoples, except for the Fulni-ô, who preserved the Iatê language. These languages were harshly repressed by Jesuits in their mission villages, but the religion could be practiced away from the priests' eyes, consecrating the beverage in silence or in rituals deep in the forest. In the missions, the jurema encantados were assimilated as local deities even by Black people, with whom Indigenous peoples had contact since the War of the Barbarians, which resulted, between 1650 and 1720, from Portuguese incursions into the semi-arid region and forced relocations to the coast.

This mixed-race population that formed in the Northeast, inheriting Indigenous traditions that converged on the ritual use of jurema, saw its cultural roots become invisible under the generic and seemingly amorphous label of "caboclos." The progressive loss of territories only began to be reversed in the 1920s, with the start of land recognition for Indigenous peoples by the Indian Protection Service (SPI). The slow process of recovering distinct identities and cultures, in which torés and the jurema cult would play an important role, gained momentum from the 1980s and culminated in the creation, in 1990, of the Articulation of Indigenous Peoples of the Northeast, Minas Gerais, and Espírito Santo (APOINME), which brings together seventy peoples distributed across 130 territories at various stages of demarcation, home to 213,000 people.[3] More than four centuries of dispossession were overturned by the 1988 Constitution, which enshrined the original right to traditional Indigenous lands and spurred the ethnic resurgence movement centered in the Northeast. As a result, in the 2022 Census, the federal statistics office IBGE identified Bahia and Pernambuco as the second and fourth states with the largest self-declared Indigenous populations, with 229,000 and 107,000 inhabitants, respectively, behind only Amazonas (491,000) and Mato Grosso do Sul (116,000).[4]

It can be said that Jurema is the first Brazilian religion, as it has the oldest records, states Salles. "It is the miracle of jurema in the face of so much persecution. The strength of the religious experience with jurema, with the beverage, is incredible and ensures its continuity." In addition to being a professor, anthropologist, and author of the book *À Sombra da Jurema Encantada*, Salles is a musician, an accomplished guitarist, and composer. One of his guitar suites is dedicated to Malunguinho, a title given to leaders of the Catucá quilombo, one of many fugitive enslaved Blacks which resisted for more than a decade in the forest of the same name, in the municipality of Abreu e Lima. The last Malunguinho is said to have been João Batista, but his lineage was immortalized as a kind of collective deity celebrated in Jurema as the Kings Malunguinho. In the same way, the plural Kings Canindé are venerated, a reminiscence of Indigenous commanders in the War of the Barbarians against the Portuguese, who, when descending into a Jurema terreiro, "radiate" everyone, with several people marking the incorporation of the entity by forming an arrowhead with their index finger and thumb. "The strength of Canindé and Malunguinho in this area of Paraíba is indisputable," says Salles, referring to the city of Alhandra.

In the anthropologist's view, it is very difficult to trace a linear history of religion in Brazil: "Traditions feed on rupture. The search for purity leads to a dead end," he says, criticizing the view that sees degeneration in the presence of African elements in the religiosity of Indigenous origin that would become known (and persecuted) as Catimbó, lately renamed as Jurema Sagrada. "Jurema masters are not concerned with being faithful to an academic category."

On the same trip in which I participated as a subject in the pilot experiment with DMT at the IC/UFRN, in Natal (see Chap. 1), I rented a car to drive to Baía da Traição, in Paraíba, where I had arranged to meet the shaman Isaias Marculino da Silva, known as Guarapirá, on May 16, 2022. We met in the tree-filled backyard of his home in the Potiguara Indigenous Land, where I interviewed him about the efforts to revive, or rather, reinvent, the traditional practices of his people. At the heart of this endeavor is the Full Moon Ritual, which we headed to after our conversation.

Then 34 years old, Guarapirá arrived already painted at the Pau-Ferro grove, an island of trees in a sea of sugarcane surrounding the Indigenous territory.[5] In the trunk of the rental car were drums, pipes, a large bottle of jurema wine, a feather headdress, and a skirt made of embira fibers. On this Monday, the ritual was held once again, as it has been every month since 2013. Isaias addressed about thirty participants and explained that the person being honored that night was Pajé Chico, the oldest shaman in the region, who had died five days earlier at the age of 76: "He is no longer with us in body, but in spirit." He said that he was not simply buried, but planted in the earth, changing planes to strengthen the trunk of the Potiguara—a metaphor among many related to trees that flourish among jurema practitioners.

The shaman gives thanks to Father Tupã, to the enchanted beings, and to the ancestors, as well as to everyone present, especially Seu Tonhô, 88 years old, companion of the late Chico in the struggles for the "retomada," the name given by the reemerged indigenous peoples of the Northeast to the fight for land recovery. In his opening speech for the ceremony, he explains that the Full Moon Ritual is a reunion of generations, regardless of a person's beliefs, an Indigenous ritual that provides guidance, that opens space for the ancestors of all:

> The confusion of the [Covid] pandemic greatly affected everyone's psychological state. The Full Moon Ritual is also about this: strengthening oneself psychologically and spiritually. We believe that within a psychological problem there is a spiritual problem. When we treat ourselves spiritually, we become stronger and can endure the suffering of daily life, the struggle. That is why one cannot live without spirituality, regardless of religion, color, or belief. Here, there is an exchange of energy, of spirituality. Here, we are all equal, we are brothers and sisters, each with their own faith, in a ritual of surrender. Do not fear these energies; here, no one is alone or abandoned.

The so-called "Jurema table," despite its name, is set on the ground. There are lit candles, the ceremonial drink, pipes (one of them with several mouthpieces stuck into the same bowl), a ceramic plate with tobacco, and maracás. To the right, a group of women dressed in embira fiber skirts settle into plastic chairs. One of Isaias's sons, Iakarynauê, ten years old, also wears a fiber skirt like his father.

Unlike this coastal group, the inland ethnicities usually keep their ceremonies closed to non-Indigenous people, such as the retreat called Ouricuri by the Fulni-ô people. This is not the case with the Potiguara, who open their Full Moon Ritual to anyone who wishes to attend. A van from the Federal University of Paraíba (UFPB) arrives with students brought by Lusival Antonio Barcellos, a professor of religious studies. Among the group is Surama Santos Ismael da Costa, a mathematician who, three weeks later, would defend a doctoral thesis on this very ritual at the UFPB,[6] supervised by Barcellos (who also supervises Isaias's master's degree). Surama explains that the utterance incomprehensible to the journalist is the Lord's Prayer in the Indigenous language Tupi-Guarani:

> *Oré rub, ybákype tekoar*
> *I moetepýramo nde rera t'oîkó*
> *T'our nde Reino!*
> *T'onhemonhang nde remimotara ybype*
> *Ybákype i nhemonhanga îabé!*
> *Oré remi'u, 'ara îabi'ondûara, eîme'eng kori orébe.*
> *Nde nhyró oré angaîpaba resé orébe, oré rerekomemûãsara supé oré nhyrõ iabé.*

The fire is lit, and the ritual opens with the gaita, a type of gourd flute whose sound is reminiscent of the fifes of Northeastern Brazil. The opening chant is initiated by the pajé, and the verses are then repeated by the others. "Who painted the fine pottery / Was the Flower of Wonder / Father and Son and Holy Spirit / Son of the Virgin Mary," goes one of them. The drink prepared by Isaias is served, made with white jurema, cold water, wine, honey, leaves, bark, roots or seeds of jurema, and other plants that are not disclosed: "It's a pajé's secret." He cannot say whether the drink was originally used by the Potiguara, but he affirms that the ceremonial use has been practiced for decades by his people—centuries, he corrects himself. Each visitor receives about one hundred milliliters of the beverage they call wine, half a disposable plastic cup, a measure imposed by the pandemic (previously, the same bowl was used for everyone). Only the pajé, the elders, and the initiates drink the beverage several times throughout the ceremony. The taste is vegetal, sweet, and alcoholic, reminiscent of jenipapo liqueur offered by Dona Raquel in Alhandra. The psychedelic effect is absent, as the pajé warns. "There's no hallucinogen, but there is energy," assures Isaias. "It's a portal of permission for spirituality. If you allow it, it will open a portal for greater concentration, but it also depends a lot on the person and the occasion." In the dissertation resulting from four years of involvement with the ritual, Surama da Costa describes the effect the drink had on her[7]:

> After the third bowl of jurema, peace reigned within me. He [Isaias] bowed at my feet and began the fumigation ritual. I was afraid I would feel unwell from the smoke, but to my surprise, as the caboclo [incorporated by the pajé] blew his pipe, placing his mouth at the opening of the oven, on the side opposite to where one usually smokes, his smoke sharpened my senses as it enveloped my body.
> I smelled the wonderful aroma of burning herbs, I heard the sound of the maracá more intensely and clearly, and I tasted even more the sweet flavor of jurema in my mouth. My body trembled. With no strength in my legs, I fell to my knees on the ground. At that moment, I felt an explosion in my heart, which began to beat at a rapid pace, incompatible with the calm that inhabited me. (Author's translation with the help of artificial intelligence)

The ceremony continues with several chants until ten at night, invoking Jurema, various other caboclos, and Oxóssi, an African deity.

> *I call the feathered cabocas, I called her to come help us*
> *Where is the strength of Jurema, where is the strength that Jurema gives*
> *Oh feathered caboca, oh feathered caboca, have mercy on me, have pity*

Some participants dance in a circle around the table, surrounded by trees, moving counterclockwise, stomping their bare feet on the ground, while others keep the rhythm with maracás. Besides Isaias and one of the elders, three Black women enter into trance and receive spirits. The first to incorporate an entity is Dona Rosa, who appears to be over seventy years old and was described by Guarapirá as an "old Indian woman" who drank jurema without any issues of interference with continuous-use medications. Bent over herself, the healer "for more than forty years" keeps one hand on her forehead and the other on her back, uttering grunts and sounds that sometimes resemble animal vocalizations.

Still at the pajé's house, before we headed into the forest, she recounted that she had received from God the gift of healing, for which she has never charged: "The word of God is not for sale. I see, I ask my gypsy," she says, referring to a class of entities venerated in Umbanda and also common in Jurema Sagrada sessions alongside masters, old Black spirits, cowboys, and sailors. She also says that she was "crazy" and was hospitalized in a psychiatric colony in João Pessoa, from which she claims to have left worse than she entered:

I was beautiful, gorgeous, I came back suru [said of animals without a tail or with a docked tail], my hair reached my buttocks. Daughter of Oxum, of Xangô, of Cabocla Iracema. It was a doctor [from the city] of Rio Tinto who discovered [my mediumship]. On February 5th, it will be forty years since I left. Now I can say that I am free, wonderful, I have my gift, my jurema, and my saint.

The moon shines through the leaves of the pau-ferro trees. The last two incorporations take hold of Tonhô and Guarapirá after several sips of jurema. The pajé, increasingly hoarse and sweaty, commands the terreiro. Toward the end of the ceremony, one of the seated women invites anyone who wishes to consult with the Caboclo of the Sacred Forests manifested by Guarapirá. A long line forms. One by one, people kneel before the enchanted being. The caboclo conveys messages to them in an inaudible voice, touches their shoulders, head, or chest, enveloping them in thick smoke rising from the pipe stem as he blows through the bowl. Once the Jurema table is closed, again after a gaita note, everyone sings:

The caboclo from the village, when he goes to the sea to fish
From his hair he makes the thread, from the thread he makes the landuá
The caboclos in the village sifting the sand[8]

After the ritual, the group proceeds to the shaman's house in the Lagoa do Mato village. A supper of tapioca, rice, and fish is served in plastic bowls, in an atmosphere of joy and communion. Two police officers from the Paraíba Indigenous Patrol share the meal. The detachment was created, it is said, to provide security for 32 Potiguara villages in the cities of Baía da Traição, Rio Tinto, and Marcação. It was not always this way. The white man's police, both before and after the ethnic group's official recognition in 1930, were almost always on the side of the sugarcane plantation owners who invaded their lands. Although they had already received from Brazilian emperor Dom Pedro II the grant of the areas they occupied, the legal recognition of their land would drag on until 1991, when 21,000 hectares of the Potiguara Indigenous Land were officially demarcated, where about 15,000 people lived in 2010, according to federal health foundation Funasa records.[9]

Isaias says he heard his calling in a dream. He was under a tree that seemed like a cave: "It was truly a revelation, the ancestors speaking to me. It was a ritual of Indians from the past and present, saddened by the weakened spirituality of the Potiguara. They said someone was needed to revive these rituals." The Caboclo of the Virgin Forest and the Cabocla of Oxóssi of the Jurema summoned him to seek the strength of the enchanted beings to uplift the Potiguara and continue the struggle with determination. Guarapirá then dedicated himself to study on two fronts. With elder shamans, such as the late Chico, he learned the science of jurema: how to prepare the wine, where to find and use power plants, the strength of pipes, drums, and maracás. At university, he earned a degree in pedagogy. He studied the old Tupi to teach the language and is now pursuing a master's in Religious Studies at the UFPB. The teacher runs the municipal primary school Celina Freire Rodrigues in the neighboring village of Cumaru, which has about eighty pupils. He also teaches Tupi at the state Indigenous high school Angelita Bezerra, in the Silva de Belém village, municipality of Rio Tinto, which has two hundred students.

"The spiritual ritual must go on," he says, though he rejects the label of Catimbó or Sacred Jurema, even with songs for orixás and saints. "It is a ritual unique to the Potiguara, but it is shaped by this cultural blending. We adapted. There is this mixture, but it is our ritual for empowerment. The people had to adapt and reinvent themselves in order to survive."

Secrecy, syncretism, and resistance: these are the ingredients of the sap that rises from the roots of the jurema and gives strength to the Indigenous trunk of the northeastern population, preventing it from being entirely swept away by the storm of Catholic colonization. It branched out and flourished into the twenty-first century, but Christianity would continue to pursue it.

Fulni-Ô, the Only Ethnic Group in the Semi-Arid Region to Keep Their Own Language Alive

In my search to learn about the still-living origins of religiosity surrounding the jurema, I made another stop—one that would prove all too brief—in Águas Belas, Pernambuco. With its 41,548 inhabitants, according to the 2022 Census, the municipality has 99.6% of its territory within the Fulni-ô Indigenous Land, where 26,300 people live (some of them in Itaíba, another municipality in Pernambuco that overlaps with the reserve). It was almost obligatory to visit the Indigenous people who managed not only to survive in a town that engulfed them since colonial times, but also to preserve their own language, Iatê, the only native language to endure in the northeastern backlands.

It would not be an exaggeration to say that, without the black jurema, the process of ethnic reemergence of the indigenous peoples of the Northeast— especially those who resisted the genocidal incursions of European colonizers in the backlands—would not have occurred. The beverage prepared from the root of this typical caatinga tree still occupies the center of the rituals of many of these peoples, always surrounded by secrets, such as those that protect the preparation of the potion which, according to accounts from the eighteenth century, fills their minds with visions of enchanted beings living in other worlds and realms inaccessible to outsiders. The most eloquent example of this strategy is offered by the Fulni-ô themselves, a group that spends part of the year secluded in forest villages where non-Indigenous people are not welcome at ceremonies.

Thus, it made sense to turn to the Fulni-ô in an attempt to pick up the thread of the jurema from the backlands, but my endeavor to uncover the uses of this tree with psychedelic powers would be neither the first nor the last to run up against a wall.

The secret lies at the heart of the Ouricuri, the most important ritual of this Iatê-speaking ethnic group—a melodious language, full of vowels, classified within the Macro-Jê stock, though it fits into none of its families. For about fourteen weeks, between August and December, many Fulni-ô families living in the urban area of Águas Belas withdraw to a separate village where outsiders are only admitted to the opening celebration and are then asked to leave the ceremonial camp. There, they perform songs, dances, and rituals with jurema about which all members of the people are forbidden to speak, under penalty of illness and death for the indiscreet. Ouricuri is the name of a palm tree whose fronds were once used to build the huts of the temporary village in the forest, but nowadays, according to accounts I heard, there are permanent masonry dwellings. The name also refers to the palm's small fruit, much prized in the region.

The Fulni-ô currently hold 12,000 hectares of land reserved in 1926 by the SPI,[10] the predecessor of the National Foundation for Indigenous Peoples (Funai), created in 1910 by Cândido Mariano Rondon. As of 2024, the territory still lacked federal ratification. It is possible to walk the short distance from the main square of Águas Belas to the village, passing through a gateway shaped like a stylized headdress with red, blue, green, and yellow feathers marking the entrance to the indigenous neighborhood. The main street leads to the square where the municipal school and the church, decorated with indigenous motifs and dedicated to Our Lady of the Immaculate Conception, are located. A few more minutes and the cluster of poor houses on dirt roads gives way to a series of small farms, one of which contains the three huts where I would have a brief glimpse of Fulni-ô culture, guided by the teacher Rangel Lúcio de Matos, known as Gel, whose name in his language is Ytoá.

At the time of this visit, in the first days of December 2022, the Ouricuri retreat was underway, already nearing its end. Normally, only those indigenous people with steady jobs in Águas Belas, like Ytoá, would be allowed to leave the ritual. Employed by the city as a doorman at the school in the permanent village, he also works as a teacher of Iatê. A student of anthropologist Sandro de Salles at the UFPE in Caruaru, where he studies intercultural literature, Ytoá agreed to guide me on a brief visit to the Indigenous land adjacent to the town.

Three other Fulni-ô interrupted the retreat for about an hour in order to meet me: the elder Xixiá and the young men Feá and Thulny. They made a pragmatic exception for the journalist, interested in establishing contact with someone from the Southeast who could help them find ways to extend their occasional "vivências" (as they call the paid presentations they give outside the villages, for non-indigenous audiences) to São Paulo and other cities. But Fulni-ô hospitality has a clear limit; it does not include an invitation to visit the Ouricuri village or to penetrate the mysteries of their jurema rituals.

At 73, revered by the other three Fulni-ô present, Xixiá does not fit the stereotype of an Indigenous person held by people from the Southeast. Fair-skinned, wearing thick-rimmed glasses with strong lenses, a sleeveless blue T-shirt, and a straw hat with a ribbon around the short brim, he could easily be mistaken for a veteran samba musician from Rio de Janeiro. Seated in the wattle-and-daub and thatch hut on a mattress without sheets, he is transformed when he intones, to the rhythm of the maracá in his right hand, one of the Iatê chants he says he receives directly from sacred beings of light, the guardians of the forest. Lying in a hammock, Feá explains: "Now we are taking his place." Both smoke pipes constantly, one of them with a colored mouthpiece and bowl. The other, conical and stemless, has a more traditional appearance and is known in the northeastern backlands as campiô; Xixiá wields it with authority. His brother was João Pontes, the chief who founded the bilingual Iatê school and led the Fulni-ô for six decades until his death at 93 in 2018, revered for his serenity and determination to resolve disputes peacefully.[11]

"Fulni-ô do not use jurema for harm, but there are outsiders who use it to do evil," Xixiá says simply. "Only for good," adds Feá, "not to interfere in anyone's life or harm anyone. If a person has a being of light, like Cacique Pena Branca, and does not know how to guide it, we give jurema so they can learn to guide it." This reference to the caboclo entity of the urban religions Jurema Sagrada and Umbanda does not clash with indigenous identity, for anyone who studies these religions and the spirituality of the Northeast's ethnic groups soon learns that there is no purity or impermeability in any of these cultural formations—quite the opposite.

The explanation continues with Ytoá: "[When there is a] house with negative energy, jurema is used to cleanse that person. Anxiety, depression is also [very] closely connected to the spirit. To drive away what is bad." The healing performed by shamans, however, is reserved for those of the same ethnicity, "within the community." Those who travel to bring jurema to the cities are the "warriors" like Feá, who was scheduled to travel in ten days to Fortaleza, capital city of the Ceará state where he would lead a ceremony alongside an Indigenous brother from the Amazon responsible for serving ayahuasca. These forays into urban territory serve to supplement income and support Fulni-ô families, which used to be done by gathering resources from nature. "Our game is extinct," Feá explains, "we went five, six years without rain. We have to go hunt outside our village, in Brasília, Rio de Janeiro, and São Paulo. Present our sacred medicine, perform healing rituals, cures."

Ytoá does not take part in these trips to the capitals, but he often travels to Caruaru, 180 km from Águas Belas, where he is pursuing an intercultural teaching degree. This is the prerequisite for being officially hired as a teacher, a role he already fulfills by teaching the Iatê language. Until his professional goal is achieved, he supplements his income with occasional construction work and also describes himself as a writer (he has plans for two novels), a poet (writing song lyrics), and a musician (he plays guitar and drums).

The melody sung by Xixiá sounds calm, almost melancholic. These are tunes that have been given the enigmatic Portuguese name "cafurna," meaning something like a hiding place, from which the verb "encafurnar" (to hide away) is derived. The young people join in chorus when the verse repeats. At the end of the brief gathering, it is Thulny, the only one dressed in traditional attire, who sings two equally gentle cafurnas, the last one to bless the visitor. Ytoá harmonizes, perfectly in tune. Without understanding a word of what they sing in Iatê, my eyes well up, overcome by an emotion hard to explain; I thank them deeply at the end, from the heart. Perhaps it was simply the satisfaction of experiencing "Indigeneity," as idealized as it was unexpected, in that hut. Despite its brevity, I choose to believe that a true encounter, or exchange, as the hosts repeatedly say, took place—even in the face of withheld information about the Ouricuri and jurema that I sought. I feel that to press further with questions would be to forgo participating in that moment of communion, freely offered to me.

Thulny sets aside Iatê and explains in Portuguese, though in a cryptic way, how his ancestors are said to have learned to prepare the infusion: "An elder wanted to have vision beyond sight and made this medicine to drink at night and have the vision of the ancestors from where she came, to bring the strength of nature," summarizes the young man in black shorts, his face and chest covered in black paint with arrow-like designs, wearing a kind of yellow-feathered headdress, a necklace of animal teeth, and a maracá made from a gourd in his right hand—the same hand that wears a large black plastic electronic watch.

"Jurema, she is a mother, she is nurturing. A medicine for healing, cleansing, and strength for our spirit." While Thulny speaks in Portuguese, Xixiá, in his own language, seems to be giving instructions about what the young man should or should not say. The young man continues: "She brings the strength of Mother Earth, this energy is always around us." They exchange a few words in Iatê, and the four Indigenous people laugh; I ask why. My guide, Ytoá, replies that laughter is a way to breathe: "When we talk about spirituality, about the sacred, we can't take it too seriously, because it is so ancient." He explains: "We can't go too deep, that's why we laugh. Jurema is like a portal between the material and the immaterial. You have to be very careful. There can be great harm, mentally. You might leave the material reality and risk not coming back."

As can be seen, it is not at all easy to obtain straightforward information about the Fulni-ô, much less about the drink made from black jurema, which is occasionally served to non-Indigenous people in ceremonies across Brazil. Despite the secrecy carefully maintained by members of the group, the answer is supplemented in Iatê by Feá, with Ytoá translating: "Jurema is similar to ayahuasca, we prepare it, but we don't add much inhibitor, because [the white person] might not return to earth. We lower the dosage, to open the path for healing, both material and spiritual." In these cases, he says, they use the bark of the caatinga tree trunk, not the root's inner bark, which would have more natural inhibitor: "When it's made from the root, the visions are stronger."

Ytoá invited me to lunch the next day at his house in the urban village, during another break from the Ouricuri retreat, which made me suspect that adherence to the custom is not as strict as claimed. Married to Luciana, who prepares the food while holding a rustic long-stemmed pipe in her mouth, he has a twelve-year-old daughter, Vivian, who is training to become a singer. The father asks her to turn off the TV where cartoons from the Cartoon Network channel are playing. He picks up the guitar and turns on the karaoke microphones. He sings sertanejo (Brazilian country music) hits with the girl, supporting her with harmonies in the choruses. The performance reaches its peak of eclecticism when the bespectacled girl sings, with a deep and powerful voice, the song *Hallelujah* by the Canadian (and Buddhist) Leonard Cohen, but in a free version in the Iatê language. As if to confirm the line from the original English lyrics that says there is a blaze of light in every word, the scene dazzles the eyes with a spark of emotion:

> *Sathawasêy djaka ookê,*
> *Saskê ywakêlha-netê yassatholha-afênkya fássatê.*
> *Saf'sêênêsse êdwalhaskê, tha fytxôlha yatxyhãnkya-hê.*
> *Eedjadwalha doowsêy yôôhê lwlya*
> *Yôôhê lwlya, yôôhê lwlya, yôôhê lwlya.*

The father then explains that the words in his version in the Indigenous language have a pedagogical purpose. It is a father's exhortation to his children, lamenting that they and their friends do not speak Iatê, since the things of non-Indigenous people seem more captivating to them, such as cell phone videos. In the song's lyrics, the father warns that by following this path, they will cease to be Fulni-ô:

> *Once again, I am here to tell you that there must be respect among us.*
> *We are failing to unite; this way, we will be lost in paradise.*
> *Without God, we are small (few)…*
> *We are small (few)*
> *We are small (few).*

Luciana interrupts the singing to announce that lunch is ready. Ytoá talks about the books he intends to write, whose drafts he keeps on a hard drive: *Fulni-ô: Nativos do Brasil* and *José de Todo Mundo*. He says he likes to reflect on humanity and history. He writes poems, which come to him even at night, and sometimes entire songs. "I've lost a lot because I didn't have paper or a recorder at hand," he says, alluding to my visible tools.

He then offers a "soul brother's advice" about the rushed visit, which would end in the afternoon with a return trip to Recife: "Those who rush grow weary; those who walk go further." He says he fears that my profession might prevent me from being myself, more than just a journalist, and states that, in his case, it does not matter where he is—he feels at home because he knows he will return and find refuge in the Ouricuri. He then asks his daughter to bring him the chanduca, a handcrafted pipe carved from the tough wood of the aroeira tree, so we can smoke in the hammocks after lunch, in another moment of communion and peace.

The hospitality of the Fulni-ô excludes the rural village space where they retreat for the Ouricuri, and the only exception occurs on the morning when the ritual retreat begins, when a Catholic mass is held at the camp, in which non-Indigenous people are accepted. The anthropologist Miguel Colaço Bittencourt, who lived in the area for several months for his doctoral research at the UFPE,[12] reports that he obtained much information about the way of life and customs of this people, such as the use of so-called "búzios" (a type of flute with a horn-like sound) in the torés, but that he was invited to leave the community when he began asking questions about the Pig clan, one of the family groups with common ancestors into which this Indigenous society is divided—in this case, the clan traditionally responsible for serving jurema at the Ouricuri. He would return to the area several times after that. It was not, in fact, a banishment, but rather a clarification of the boundaries between what is shown to outsiders and what belongs to the Indigenous people and their secrets: "The Ouricuri can be seen as a classroom that teaches a time and a way of being Indigenous in the Northeast, a ritual school where a sense of 'us' and 'I' is socialized in the same symbolic action," Bittencourt wrote in his thesis.

Familiar with ayahuasca since the age of seventeen, Bittencourt also explored what some neo-shamans call "juremahuasca." He became interested in jurema as a research topic and, in 2016, began his doctorate with Edwin Reesink at the UFPE, which he completed in 2022. During the periods he lived in the village, he witnessed some "torés de búzios" performed for non-Indigenous people, concluding that this practice offers a kind of summary of the toré held during the Ouricuri, to which outsiders have no access. There are older ethnographic accounts—such as that of Estêvão Pinto, one of the first scholars to gather information about this people in the 1940s—but the Fulni-ô say it is all untrue, projecting onto the distant past the strict secrecy they developed through a long history of domination and pressure against their culture and lands.

This conflicted contact with Europeans and their descendants was not without cultural assimilation and adaptation, of course. Bittencourt says that the cafurnas themselves, traditional songs of this people, were an innovation introduced in the 1970s by none other than the elder Xixiá, melodies to which the elder leader gave the Iatê name "unakesa." Today, the cafurnas are a crucial element of experiences—alongside handicrafts, incense rituals, prayers, and a non-psychedelic jurema tea—offered for non-Indigenous tourists in Águas Belas and also during trips to large cities. Another adaptation in the performances appears with the use of feather headdresses, which the Fulni-ô learned to make with the Kayapó from the Amazon at Indigenous peoples' gatherings, as previously they used only the *aloá*, a type of straw hat made from the ouricuri palm, and the caroá fiber bag they call *aió*. On some occasions, the búzios that are played are made from PVC pipes. The cafurnas have also become objects of alliance and exchange with another people of the region, the Xucuru, to whom they taught the songs; they are the only members of another culture whom the Fulni-ô allow into their Ouricuri retreat.

The main public event in the village of Águas Belas is the Festa da Santa, a tribute by the Indigenous people to Our Lady of the Immaculate Conception, held in the square of the church dedicated to her. The Fulni-ô know her as Yasakhlane, and she occupies the ambiguous position of patroness of cultural contact. According to the story told by the guide Ytoá, the image of the saint was found by Indigenous people, who are said to have broken a finger off the statue to make sure it was not alive. Bittencourt's doctoral thesis presents a less miraculous version, recounted to him by Xixiá, regarding the discovery of the image by the Indigenous people: in reality, the elder says, the wooden statue, rather than being found by chance, was repeatedly hidden in a lagoon to be found by the natives. The colonizers then spread the message that the saint wanted the Indigenous people to donate land for the construction of the temple. This is precisely what would happen in 1832, forty-five years after the parish of Our Lady of the Immaculate Conception of Águas Belas was established, a village that arose after the dissolution of the missionary settlement to which the Fulni-ô ancestors had been reduced.

Between 1876 and 1878, 11,506 hectares were demarcated for the Fulni-ô, and eighty hectares were reserved for the church and the town that had grown up around it. The Indigenous area was known as Ipanema village, named after the nearby river. In the 1920s, the recognition of Indigenous reserves by the SPI advanced in the Northeast, for which caboclo descendants of the former Indigenous people had to provide proof of Indigeneity, such as performing torés (which in the Iatê language, lacking the sound for "r," is pronounced *tolê*). This was followed by a long period of disputes over land rights, with the city of Águas Belas and leaseholders encroaching on ever larger portions of Indigenous territory, which to this day has not received definitive recognition of the 11,572 hectares established in later surveys,[13] which the Fulni-ô seek to have expanded to 57,000 hectares.

"This is a society of scarce resources, which needs innovation and creativity to achieve quality of life," explains Bittencourt. "White people arrive with the expectation of seeing the original Indians, who have no phones and live in straw huts. When they see an Indian painting himself using a cell phone [as a mirror], it is as if there is a rupture of 'spirituality'." The tourist toré, therefore, serves to demonstrate that there are living Indigenous people in Águas Belas, while the Ouricuri serves to sustain and internally reproduce their own "Indigeneity," insofar as it helps preserve the language—for a person born to a mother of the ethnicity to be recognized as Fulni-ô, they must observe the

Ouricuri, speak at least rudimentary Iatê, and, above all, maintain secrecy, under penalty of falling ill and dying. According to Bittencourt,

> [the] *secret* has become, in the Indigenous Northeast, the symbol of maintaining the boundary of ethnic identity, which is constituted by a sacred and religious universe. In this way, religion exerts great political influence. For the "secret" is invoked to express an ancestral boundary in which it is asserted that the Indians are the owners of the land.[14] (Author's translation with the help of artificial intelligence)

And, alongside the secret, certain trees emerge as markers of a cosmology and an intimacy with the land's nature that are impermeable to European religion, even when enveloped in syncretism, as the author notes: "In Northeastern Amerindian thought, if Jesus was born in a jurema tree, Our Lady of the Immaculate Conception stood before the juazeiro, and Saint Peter approached the baraúna." For the scholar, plant thought is a trait of pre-Cabralian Amerindian continuity in the understanding of descent lineages and in ritual operations to maintain bonds of origin and population grouping. In this sense, jurema, ouricuri, juazeiro, and other native plants hold a primordial position in the Northeast, serving as instruments and vehicles for access to the enchanted realm, the raw material for the drink of the enchanted beings, which cures ills and misfortunes brought by colonization.

Flexibility, Herbs, and Secrecy: Weapons Against the Colonizer

Secrecy, jurema, pipe, and maracá form a complex ideological-religious among Indigenous peoples of the Northeast, not limited to the Fulni-ô. These are cultural traits common to the peoples of the semi-arid region, where the jurema-preta flourishes, which later spread to "zona da mata," the rainforest strip along the coast, to the point of becoming almost universal in the region. Such widespread diffusion stems from the fact that this set of practices gradually acquired the character of a nucleus of resistance to Portuguese colonization, even as it assimilated European religious elements in a continuous process of syncretism that would extend into the twentieth and twenty-first centuries.

Colonized, exterminated or nearly extinct, enslaved, catechized, dispossessed, subjugated, discriminated against, mixed, acculturated, civilized—the Indigenous peoples of the Northeast "made the science of jurema withstand all of this, and their Indigeneity is today immortalized in the most diverse jurema-based religious traditions," argues anthropologist Rodrigo Grünewald,[15] perhaps the most prolific author of works on Jurema. As is evident in the case of the Fulni-ô, for whom the Ouricuri is intertwined with the cult of Our Lady of the Conception, the paradoxical blend of secrecy and assimilation has marked the cultural survival of the Indigenous peoples of the Northeast, centered on the plant, the wine, and the spirituality of Jurema, while also linking them to a strategy with deep historical roots.

Religious miscegenation, so to speak, had already begun in the 1500s, long before jurema was mentioned in official documents of the Crown or the Inquisition. The tendency toward syncretism would seem to be the result of an inherent malleability among Amerindians, whose populations were always characterized by large migrations, wars, and interethnic contacts, with oral transmission of customs that left little room for the establishment of dogmas. The adaptive capacity of Indigenous peoples was noted by anthropologist Eduardo Viveiros de Castro in a classic article, "O mármore e a murta" ("The Marble and the Myrtle"),[16] an image he drew from Antônio Vieira's 1657 "Sermon of the Holy Spirit," in which the priest compares Indigenous religiosity to those statues sculpted by pruning shrubs, often in the shape of animals: "[…] easier to shape, given the flexibility of the branches, but it is necessary to keep constantly reforming and working on it, so that it is preserved." European faith, on the other hand, corresponds to sculpture in marble, which, "once made, needs no further touch: it always maintains and sustains the same form."

What in Vieira is a vegetal metaphor for the shifting Amerindian spirituality stands in contrast to what, for the Indigenous peoples of the Northeast, is embodied in the very trees themselves, with the jurema-preta being a fitting example. Not by coincidence, the wood of the jurema is hard and full of thorns: trunk and roots that provide access to what belongs to the earth and draw from it the blood of ancestors (and even of Jesus, as would later be enshrined in the syncretic potpourri). The ingestion of jurema wine grants access to these deified dead, to the source from which colonized peoples draw strength to resist catechization, even while apparently submitting to it. The propensity to assimilate foreign elements led Jesuits to seek correspondences in native cosmologies to instill Catholic faith in those they attracted to the missions, for example by translating their own monotheistic God as Tupã. Thus, the door was opened to "believe without faith," as interpreted by Viveiros de Castro, the "mixture of volatility and obstinacy, docility and recalcitrance, enthusiasm and indifference with which the Tupinambá received the good news."

This duplicity noted by the anthropologist had already been observed in 1951 by folklorist Luís da Câmara Cascudo, who explained that the expression "adjunto de jurema," used by Jesuits and inquisitors to condemn Indigenous magic, referred to ephemeral gatherings and rituals in which the beverage was consumed:

> The Indigenous people, catechized on the outside, retained their beliefs on the inside. And, whenever possible, they practiced the forbidden ritual, dancing the Jurupari dance [an entity associated with evil] to the sound of maracás and the rumble of sacred instruments that brought death to curious women.. (Author's translation with the help of artificial intelligence)

They made the beverage with jurema and drank it in ceremonies that left no trace, he adds: "It was medicine, joy, relief, and sublimation. They drank, dreamed, and loved. Everyone thinks the festivities were worth the unheard-of daring of their clandestine realization."[17]

The ambiguous encounter between Amerindian and Christian worlds in the sixteenth century gave rise to an Indigenous phenomenon that would become known by the generic term "santidades" ("sanctities"), whose first manifestations were recorded, according to Ronaldo Vainfas, by chroniclers such as Hans Staden in 1557, André Thevet in 1558, and Jean de Léry in 1578.[18] Despite the paradoxical name, the santidades were more commonly described by Jesuit priests as heretical sects, arising from migrations and escapes from Jesuit missionary settlements, generally led by by caraíbas, itinerant superior shamans who acted as prophets or holy men among the Tupinambá, traveling from village to village making predictions or rallying their peers to set out in search of the Land Without Evil. Their preaching directly challenged the religious authority of the Europeans, claiming for themselves the status of saints, which they denied to the white enslavers and catechists, against whom they rose up in what Vainfas called "insurgent idolatries, collective acts of symbolic and social rejection of colonialism."

One of the most famous cases, and the central focus of Vainfas's book, was the Santidade of Jaguaripe, in the southern part of the Recôncavo Baiano, which is richly documented in the records produced during the First Visitation of the Holy Office of Lisbon to the Northeast (1591–1595). In the 1580s, a caraíba baptized as Antônio by the Jesuits, who had escaped from the Tinharé mission in the captaincy of Ilhéus, began to lead or inspire several revolts of captive Indigenous people on plantations in the Recôncavo, who took refuge in the forests at a place known as Palmeiras Compridas. Two expeditions were organized to find this kind of Indigenous quilombo rooted in syncretic religiosity: one official, led by Governor Teles Barreto, with the mission to destroy the santidade, and another private, initiated by the landowner Fernão Cabral. The second expedition, led by a mameluco (mixed race) named Tomacaúna, located the headquarters of the Indigenous revolt and, instead of destroying it, managed to bring an uncertain number of rebels (between sixty and two hundred, according to varying reports to the Inquisition) to Cabral's sugar mill. Among those brought were a Tupi prophetess, the caraíba known as Santa Maria or Mother of God, and a stone idol they venerated, but not the leader Antônio, who had fled.

In practice, the santidade merely relocated to the plantation; it did not disappear. The Indigenous people built a church on the property and began working for Fernão Cabral, suggesting that the purpose of the expedition led by Tomacaúna was never to suppress the revolt. The plantation owner provided material support to the sect, and his wife, Dona Margarida da Costa, became close to the women involved, taking them in as servants in her household—evidence that the pragmatic openness of the natives to foreign religion found a counterpart among the Europeans. Enslaved Indigenous people who had escaped from other properties found shelter and work there, increasing the labor force available to the mill. The outrage of other landowners at Cabral's prosperity, which grew at their expense as he enriched himself with the labor of fugitives from other plantations, led Governor Teles Barreto to send the inquisitor Bernaldim Ribeiro to put an end to the "idolatry," which he did by destroying the santidade's temple on the plantation and the idol enthroned there. Even though he was indicted and imprisoned for a year by the Holy Office, at the behest of the envoy Heitor Furtado de Mendonça, Cabral escaped with a hefty fine of one thousand cruzados (enough at the time to purchase twenty enslaved Africans) and the relatively mild punishment of two years' exile, which he served in Portugal. The visitor justified, in the sentence, that the defendant was "an Old Christian, and by his quality, nobility, and good blood, and the probability and presumed certainty that he did not harbor in his mind or spirit any internal error against the truth of our Holy Catholic Faith," as Vainfas reports.

Most of what is known about the practices of the members of the Santidade of Jaguaripe comes from the Annual Letter of 1585, probably written by José de Anchieta in the same year the church was destroyed. The rituals described as demonic there appeared alongside alleged infanticides, the myth of a ship that would come to deliver everyone from captivity, and the ubiquitous use of maracás and tobacco—though the latter was presented as a juice that the members of the santidade drank, supposedly causing the trance that overtook them. According to Vainfas, this is a mistake, since Brazilian Indigenous peoples typically smoke or fumigate with tobacco, not ingest it;

perhaps a deliberate error, intended to evoke in European readers familiar images of potions and diabolical rites. There are other possible interpretations of the references to such beverages, which could well have been cauim, a fermented drink made from plants such as manioc, or even a jurema wine that the Indigenous people may already have kept hidden from the whites—even though, in the latter case, the use of jurema-preta is less likely, since Jaguaripe was near the coast and *Mimosa tenuiflora* thrives in the inland Caatinga semi-arid biome. In any case, tobacco and jurema have remained sacred plants for the Indigenous peoples of the Northeast, playing a prominent role in efforts to reconnect with ancestors and resist colonization—a centrality that has been described as *phytolatry.*

It would take some time, however, before black jurema and the Indigenous ritual practices reminiscent of the santidades that spread throughout the Northeast in the following centuries would come under the scrutiny and records of the colonizers and their Inquisition. In the seventeenth century, there are references to ceremonies considered witchcraft, but without mentioning jurema by name, such as the 1671 account by the French priest Martinho de Nantes, who lived among the Kariri of Paraíba, cited by Luiz Assunção[19] and who refers to sorcerers or impostors who predicted future events and cured diseases. "One could believe that some of them had dealings with the Devil, for they used as remedies for all ailments nothing but tobacco smoke and certain prayers, singing tunes as wild as they, without uttering a single word." To ensure success in hunting or fishing, the masters of ceremony would give the young men "the juice of certain bitter herbs" to drink.

As described in the book *Jurema* by Rodrigo Grünewald,[20] the first mention of the jurema beverage in documents of the Holy Office dates back to 1720, when the Tabajara Jacob de Sousa e Castro traveled to Lisbon to present his people's petitions in recognition of their loyal service to the Crown and testified before the Holy Office about Indigenous people accused of drinking jurema and "summoning demons" amid the sound of maracás and the smoke of pipes. In 1739, the Overseas Missions Board in Pernambuco decided to imprison Indigenous people practicing diabolical witchcraft in the villages of Mamanguape, Paraíba (a region near Baía da Traição, where I witnessed the Potiguara Full Moon Ritual), an order that resulted in the death of a dozen natives.[21] Two years later, the governor of the captaincy of Pernambuco sent a letter to King João V referring to the imprisonment of Indigenous sorcerers:

> [...] that the necessary means be sought to remedy the errors that have taken
> root among the Indians, who are consuming certain beverages called jurema,

which leave them mad, with visions and diabolical apparitions, leading them to believe that the path taught by the missionaries is not the true one.. (Author's translation with the help of artificial intelligence)

Jesuit oversight of Indigenous people in the settlements and their near monopoly on the repression of Amerindian heresies was interrupted with the rise of the Marquis of Pombal to the position of prime minister under King José I, from 1755 to 1777. In 1757, he established the Directorate of Indians, appointing an official to oversee the Indigenous populations of Pará and Maranhão; the following year, another Directorate was created for the captaincy of Pernambuco, now with a direct prohibition, "entirely abolishing the [use] of juremas, contrary to good morals and of no benefit, but rather extremely harmful to the health of the people."[22]

The transformation of settlements under the control of the Society of Jesus into towns with civil administration continued throughout the eighteenth century, but failed to suppress the use of jurema.[23] The Jesuit missions and the towns they gave rise to, on the one hand, and the sanctities, escapes, and revolts of Indigenous and enslaved Black people fleeing from the coast to the interior, on the other, repeatedly provided opportunities for miscegenation, cultural exchange, and religious syncretism among Tupis, Tapuias, Africans, and mestizos, who spread the cult of jurema, maracás, and smoke throughout the Northeast wherever they were not already present, blending Indigenous religiosity with elements of Afro-Brazilian cults, popular Catholicism, and European magic (and later, even Kardecist Spiritism), which would give rise to Catimbó.

"Jurema and Santidade [...] are examples of these strategies of resistance, which include agreements, negotiations, and adaptations to changing cultural contexts," concludes anthropologist Sandro de Salles. Often marked by a messianic aspect, already present in the Tupi quest for the Land Without Evil, the religion/resistance binomial would survive to enter the nineteenth century with resounding revivals of the sixteenth-century sanctities.

Nearly two and a half centuries separate the Santidade of Jaguaripe from the Pedra Bonita sect, which emerged in 1836–8 in Vila Bela (Pernambuco), now the municipality of São José do Belmonte, according to a 1907 account by Francisco Pereira da Costa cited by Rodrigo Grünewald.[24] It was one of the Brazilian manifestations of Sebastianism, a prophetic movement that foretold the mystical return of the Portuguese King Sebastião I, who disappeared in 1578 at the Battle of Alcácer-Quibir in Morocco. A mestizo named João Antônio dos Santos, from the Pedra Bonita site, preached the return of the king and the time of abundance that would come with him, gaining the support of several sertanejos for his pilgrimages. Santos eventually renounced his apostolate, succumbing to the influence of a priest who convinced him of the heretical nature of the movement, but was replaced as leader of the sect by his brother-in-law João Ferreira, who proclaimed himself king and conducted rituals in a cave where he served a beverage made from jurema-preta and manacá (*Brunfelsia uniflora*).

The doctrine held that the disenchantment of the kingdom required washing the stones from the region with human and animal blood, which allegedly led to the sacrifice of thirty children, twelve men, eleven women, and fourteen dogs between May 14 and 17, 1838. This supposed massacre, in turn, prompted the extermination of the sect by a police detachment. There are doubts regarding the veracity of the alleged sacrifices, as the account was made decades later and may well have been invented to justify the massacre carried out by the police.

Grünewald notes that the Pedra Bonita region, now known as Pedra do Reino, at the tri-border area between Pernambuco, Paraíba, and Ceará, is home to several northeastern ethnic groups, such as the Xocó, Pankará, Pipipan, and Atikum. "This perspective of associating rock formations with enchanted kingdoms is very common among the Jurema-using Indigenous peoples of the region," the anthropologist observes. "Today, the entire region is marked by Jurema, enchanted kingdoms, and, it should be emphasized, violence."

Notes

1. Instituto Socioambiental, *Terras Indígenas do Brasil*. Available at: <https://terrasindigenas.org.br/pt-br/terras-indigenas/5098> . Accessed on: Aug. 25, 2023.
2. J. J. Vepsäläinen, S. Auriola, M. Tukiainen, N. Ropponen, J. C. Callaway, "Isolation and Characterization of Yuremamine, a New Phytoindole". *Planta Med*, v. 71, n. 11, pp. 1053–7, Nov. 2005. Available at: < https://doi.org/10.1055/s-2005-873131 > . Accessed on: Dec. 20, 2024.
3. Available at: <https://apoinme.org/> . Accessed on: Aug. 23, 2023.
4. Funai. Available at: <https://www.gov.br/funai/pt-br/assuntos/noticias/2023/dados-do-censo-2022-revelam-que-o-brasil-tem-1-7-mil hao-de-indigenas> . Accessed on: Aug. 25, 2023.
5. A simplified version of the following account was published on July 26, 2022, in the report "Cultos com alucinógenos da juremaflorescem no

Nordeste," the third part of the series A Ressurreição da Jurema. Available at: <https://www1.folha.uol.com.br/ilustrissima/2022/07/cultos-com-alucinogeno-da-jurema-florescem-no-nordeste.shtml> . Accessed on: Aug. 25, 2023.

6. Surama Santos Ismael da Costa, *Ritual da Lua Cheia: Espiritualidade e Tradição entre os Potiguara da Paraíba*. João Pessoa: UFPB, 2022. Doctoral thesis. Available at: <https://repositorio.ufpb.br/jspui/handle/123456789/24225> . Accessed on: Dec. 20, 2024.

7. Ibid., p. 243.

8. * Landuá is a tapered hand net used to catch small fish, like the puçá.

9. Instituto Socioambiental, *Terras Indígenas do Brasil*. Available at: <https://terrasindigenas.org.br/pt-br/terras-indigenas/3830> . Accessed on: Aug. 24, 2023.

10. Idem, *Terras Indígenas do Brasil*. Available at: <https://terrasindigenas.org.br/pt-br/terras-indigenas/3667> . Accessed on: Aug. 25, 2023.

11. Funai, "Morre um Grande Líder: Graças a ele, a cultura de seu povo permanece." Available at: https://www.gov.br/funai/pt-br/assuntos/noticias/2018/morre-um-grande-lider-mas-gracas-a-ele-sua-cultura-permanece. Accessed on: Aug. 25, 2023.

12. Miguel Colaço Bittencourt, *Fluxos de comunicação fulni-ô: Cosmologia, territorialidade e performance*. Recife: UFPE, 2022. Doctoral thesis. Available at:. Accessed on: Dec. 20, 2024.

13. Instituto Socioambiental, *Terras Indígenas do Brasil*. Available at: <https://terrasindigenas.org.br/pt-br/terras-indigenas/3667> . Accessed on: Aug. 25, 2023.

14. Miguel Colaço Bittencourt, *Fluxos de comunicação fulni-ô*.

15. Rodrigo Grünewald, *Jurema*. Campinas: Mercado de Letras, 2020. p. 255.

16. Eduardo Viveiros de Castro, "O Mármore e a Murta: Sobre a inconstância da alma selvagem" In: *A Inconstância da Alma Selvagem e Outros Ensaios de Antropologia*. São Paulo: Cosac & Naify, 2002.

17. Luís da Câmara Cascudo, *Meleagro*. Rio de Janeiro: Agir, 1978. pp. 27–8.

18. Ronaldo Vainfas, *A Heresia dos Índios*. São Paulo: Companhia das Letras, 2022. pp. 62–3.

19. Luiz Assunção, *O Reino dos Mestres*. Rio de Janeiro: Pallas, 2010.

20. Rodrigo Grünewald, *Jurema*, p. 78.

21. Alexandre L'Omi L'Odó, *Juremologia*. Recife: Catholic University of Pernambuco, 2017. Master's thesis in Social Sciences. p. 44.

22. Sandro Guimarães de Salles, *À Sombra da Jurema Encantada*. Recife: UFPE, 2010. pp. 54–5.

23. In 1788, anthropologist Sandro Guimarães de Salles notes, Father José Monteiro de Noronha published the following commentary on the Amanajó in his *Roteiro da Viagem da Cidade do Pará até as Últimas Colônias do Sertão da Província*: "Their religion is none. Among them, however, there are pitões [serpents], or sorcerers who are such only in name, pretense, and the mistaken persuasion of those who consult them for predictions of future events in which they are interested, and to whom they turn for the cure of their most stubborn illnesses. [...] In their major festivities, those most skilled in war use a drink made from the root of a certain wood called—Jurema—whose property is exceedingly narcotic." (Author's translation with the help of artificial intelligence).

24. Rodrigo Grünewald, *Jurema*, pp. 84–8.

The Sacred Jurema at the Crossroads of Catimbó and Umbanda

A mango tree and an angico tree cast their shade over the yard of Casa das Matas do Reis Malunguinho, atop the Cajueiro neighborhood in Recife. Around the trunk of the mango tree rests a row of painted wooden canes, striped in white, red, black, blue, and green. Around three in the afternoon on March 19th, St. Joseph's Day and the traditional day for planting corn in the Northeastern region of Brazil, guests begin to arrive for the Festival of the Jurema Masters and the Crab Feast for Seu Zé: many white pants, skirts, and dresses, several turbans and red blouses, floral chintz shirts. Straw hats and maracás are everywhere. In the backyard stretching to the right of the house, beyond the mango tree, stands a cross before which a "Jurema de Chão" ritual will take place, with dozens of glasses of water and candles set on the ground. On the long white wall, a red and green circle with a seven-pointed star and below it the phrase: "Here nothing is taught, but everything is learned."[1]

Those who arrive greet one another. They show special reverence to Teca de Oyá, 77 years old at the time, an Umbanda practitioner with half a century of experience and rings on every finger, a special guest of Alexandre L'Omi L'Odó, the patron of the house. Some proceed down the corridor to the left of the building, passing a white and green pot inscribed "Jurema Preta Senhora Rainha" in which a *Mimosa tenuiflora* shrub flourishes, heading toward the small room of offerings filled with plates and wooden bowls of fruit and other foods. To the right as you enter the room, a door opens to a smaller space, painted red and black, with many exu tridents and statuettes of pombajiras (respectively male and female trickster entities revered in Afro-Brazilian spirituality). On the small porch, the bare torso of a giant doll made by artist

© The Author(s), under exclusive license to Springer Nature
Switzerland AG 2026
M. Leite, *The Psychedelic Science of the Jurema Tree*, Copernicus Books,
https://doi.org/10.1007/978-3-032-22705-8_4

Sílvio Botelho depicts a strong bare-chested Black man. Teca de Oyá remarks: "That Malunguinho was a hit at Carnival."

As the sun sets, a circle forms between the mango tree and the cross, with the house's members seated on stools around the glasses and candles. They sing "Chegou agora / Chegou agora," (he just arrived) referring to Reis Malunguinho. Alexandre, wearing a straw hat with a hole in the top and a red scarf around his neck, begins to speak in a hoarse voice, already possessed by the enchanted master who gives the house its name. The disciples line up to receive his blessing. The entity drinks cachaça straight from the bottle and also from a bottle of dark liquid, which is shared with his godchildren, embracing them and speaking to each one, as if delivering "messages" (advice, recommendations): it is the jurema wine, passed from hand to hand until it reaches me; I take a sip of the sweet, herbal-tasting drink, similar to the liqueur Dona Raquel gave me in Alhandra (see Chap. 2), which I will confirm in the following hours has no psychedelic effect on me.

A young man walks backwards to the entrance gate carrying a gourd and a candle. In the street, he pours the spirit from the gourd onto the ground. He returns with the candle and places it in the small house to the left of the entrance, dedicated to Exu. Someone comes to call me to speak with Malunguinho, and I ask if I may enter the circle with my head uncovered, since everyone there is wearing a hat, and I am given a small brown felt hat, which I balance on my crown. Alexandre/Malunguinho embraces me tightly, his shirt sweaty, slightly trembling, then steps back and fumigates my body, blowing a thick jet of smoke from his pipe through the mouthpiece. He approaches, places his hand over my heart, and tells me to take care of it, without making clear whether he means the vital organ or the symbolic seat of emotions—perhaps both—and mutters something about wearing white. The brief interaction with the entity is charged with emotion; there is something genuine in that energy, in the intention and the call for healing, that challenges a journalist's skepticism.

There are at least fifty people at the celebration. The godchildren sing around the princes and princesses, glasses and goblets of water alluding to the cities of Jurema: "Hold me in the world / Sustain me / Juremá / Sustain me." Accompanied only by the sound of maracás, they sing a chant I had already heard in João Pessoa: "Jurema is an enchanted wood / A wood of science / That everyone wants to know."

The patron of the house coined the term "juremology" to designate the study of the complex mythology of the Sacred Jurema, a religion descended from Catimbó and a cousin of Umbanda. He used the neologism as the title of his master's thesis, defended in 2017 at the Federal University of

Pernambuco (UFPE), with the subtitle "An ethnographic search for the systematization of the principles of the Sacred Jurema worldview." Born Alexandre Alberto Santos de Oliveira, the author officially changed his surname to L'Omi L'Odó in 2011, a pioneer in doing so for religious reasons; he explains that the new name means "of the waters of the rivers" in Yoruba. All people of the terreiro in Pernambuco have dual belonging, he explains: they practice Jurema and Candomblé, in the regional variant known as Xangô, even if on separate days and in separate rituals. His house, however, is only for Jurema, "but one day it will also be of Candomblé."

The Oliveira family originates from the backlands of Pernambuco, near Cabrobó, with Black ancestors and roots in the Truká indigenous ethnicity, one of the twelve original peoples present in the state. These roots were denied, he says, when they moved to the coast after his grandmother's land was taken, since not identifying as indigenous was the norm: "Self-recognition is only forty years old," he explains, referring to the cultural resurgence of indigenous peoples in the Northeast. Today, Alexandre sees himself as a continuation of the family's line of shamans. He found faith at thirteen, but claims to have been born "with the science," receiving his training from Dona Leide, his godmother in Jurema. By seventeen, he was already "reading the cards."

"We really do start from the bottom," he said in an interview days before the festival, pointing to the young women and men sweeping the yard and painting the cross. "The important thing is to take care of the house, to prepare the environment for good energies. I was a boy who gathered herbs, I learned about them from her [Dona Leide]," he recounts. "They labeled Jurema as an initiatory religion. That's fake news. Jurema is an innate science, it's not initiatory like Candomblé." For him, the best juremeiras are old women who have never set foot in a terreiro like his.

The encounter that would change his life happened with the historical figure Malunguinho, until then a divinity present only in Jurema chants, such as those in which Reis Malunguinho is presented as the watchman and guardian of Jurema, the warrior of 71 battalions. It was in 2006, thanks to Hildo Leal da Rosa, historian of the Xambá terreiro and coordinator of the João Emerenciano State Public Archive in Recife. A paleographer, that is, a specialist in ancient manuscripts, Rosa helped fellow historian Marcus Carvalho transcribe nineteenth-century documents about the Catucá quilombo, a remote forested area that sheltered runaway slaves. The repeated references to Malunguinho as leader of the rebels caught the paleographer's attention, a practitioner of Afro-Brazilian cults who recognized the name from the chants he heard in the terreiros.[2]

Alexandre was still an undergraduate history student, but he knew Rosa. With him and João Monteiro, he started in 2004 a study group that would give rise to the Quilombo Cultural Malunguinho (QCM). Unlike the movement to recognize other Black refuges such as the Quilombo dos Palmares (AL), which involved archaeological studies, in this case there was only documentary history to support recognition as a cultural and religious heritage, rather than territorial. In the same year, 2006, the group organized the first Kipupa Malunguinho festival, bringing together fifty people at the site Alexandre had been directed to by a "message" from the divinity itself: heading to a property where archaeologists were excavating a possible quilombo in the rural area of the Abreu e Lima municipality, the bus broke down at a site whose owner, Juarez, was a juremeiro. They had arrived at the in Catucá Quilombo.

The festival would be repeated every year for two decades, with a growing audience until the covid-19 pandemic, when the happening shrank to fewer than a hundred people. At its peak, in 2019, it brought together thousands of participants in the forest, which was difficult to access, with twelve kilometers of dirt road along the way. The mobilization, which Alexandre, in his dissertation, called the "Catimbó Revolution" and described as an intellectual uprising,[3] led in 2017 to the adoption of State Law No. 16,241 establishing the Afro-Pernambucan Culture Week from September 12 to 18, in honor of Malunguinho. As leader of the movement, Alexandre gave a lecture in Brasília to members of the National Institute of Historic and Artistic Heritage (IPHAN) as part of the process to make Catucá and Malunguinho cultural heritage of Brazil, a process that was halted during Jair Bolsonaro's anti-quilombo presidency.

The calunga (Malunguinho giant doll), whose torso is parked on the veranda of the terreiro's headquarters, commanding the admiration of Teca de Oyá, has the unadorned appearance of a strong Black man. Its appearance at Carnival, like the Kipupa festival, crowned the resurgence of Malunguinho in the cultural world, giving visibility to a figure previously buried among forgotten papers in the archives, but very much alive in Jurema rituals and their sung chants, even if dissociated from the historical quilombo leader. It is not surprising, then, that Malunguinho is at the center of the terreiro's festival that bears his name and is incorporated by the host, godfather to all those attending.

Other mediums present also receive entities, as is the case with singer and journalist Joanah Flor, who is possessed by Cigana, a pombajira. Highly sensual, she comes down at the start of the celebration, when the drums play in a circle for Exu, with a glass of sparkling wine in one hand and a lit cigarette in the other. She came up to me, took a pipe, and began to blow a lot of smoke up and down my body, first in front and then behind, for purification. She then did the same with the camera, recorder, and notebook I was holding. She asked me to set the items aside on a bench and gather everything in my hands whatever was needed—love, certainly—and, after the smoke, would "send it out into the world" (in this case, upwards). The blessing from the entity moved me just as much as the encounter with Malunguinho through Alexandre, as would happen again on other occasions, much to the visitor's surprise, who would remain an atheist, despite everything.

At another moment during the celebration, when the ritual was Jurema de chão, Joanah incorporated her guiding entity, Mestra Luziara. The singer, whose trance involves complete possession and leaves no memory, only identified the enchanted being afterward, through a photograph I took of her during the ceremony: a serene face, delicate and discreetly smiling, in contrast to the exuberance of the dancing Cigana who had preceded her. According to a Jurema narrative, Luziara was once the lover of Dom João VI, and sought refuge in Pernambuco after the royal family returned to Portugal after his 13-year exile in Brazil (1808–1821). According to Joanah, she is considered the oldest master of Jurema, and some predict that she will stop descending from the realm of the enchanted to work in the terreiros, as several practitioners claim has already happened with Zé Pelintra, who for many has withdrawn from terreiros, although some still seem to incorporate him, such as Pai Ciriaco in Alhandra.

Joanah made a documentary about Jurema Sagrada that her godfather, Alexandre, considers one of the best audiovisual works on the religion. Entitled "Jurema Sagrada: The Science of the Enchanted,"[4] the 23-min film, produced in 2008 as her journalism graduation project at the Catholic University of Pernambuco (UNICAP), features interviews and scenes from various Jurema houses, including the ruins of Maria do Acais's site in Alhandra, of which not even traces would remain later. The singer says she did not make the documentary just to fulfill an academic requirement, but in response to a spiritual calling, "all mystical." Born into a family from eastern Maranhão state, "very catechized," she did not even know what Jurema was until she began her research for the project.

I asked Joanah for help in finding a traditional maracá made from cuité, a very round type of gourd that grows as a bright green fruit on the cuieira tree (*Crescentia cujete*). We visited several stalls at the São José market, in Recife's port area, until we found a maracá with an intense, uniform, and high-pitched rattle. The interview took place over lunch with escondidinho de bode, a goat casserole with cassava, on Rua da Guia, a famous red-light district in Recife also associated with Jurema masters, such as Ritinha, whom I met in the Redinha neighborhood of Natal. Back at the terreiro in the Cajueiro neighborhood, where the shrine room displays an old blue enamel street sign from Rua da Guia with white letters, she sang two Jurema songs, one for Cigana and another for Malunguinho (all translations of quotes, verses and lyrics from Portuguese in this chapter are the author's with help of AI):

Pay attention, young man
Don't play with women
One day you're on top
The next you're on the ground
Pay attention, young man
Watch what you do
I am Pombajira Cigana
And I have eyes behind me

How long will the sea live
How long will it survive
How long will the river run
How long will you keep smiling
Watching everything disappear
Disappear
And when the Sun burns out
And the Moon is never seen again
And you can't even breathe
You'll run, you'll flee without arriving
Anywhere, or grow tired
My love of the forest
In the seed, in the flower, in the bark
In the root of the forest
In the backlands, in the city, far from here
Sobô Nirê, Sobô Nirê
Sobô Nirê, Sobô Nirê
I fixed my point, yes
In the middle of the forest, yes
Sobô Nirê, Sobô Nirê
Sobô Nirê, Sobô Nirê
Malunguinho in the forest is King
Malunguinho in the forest is King

The Amerindian and Afro-Brazilian Ancestors Preceding Umbanda

The presence of Zé Pelintra in Jurema rituals, as well as exus, pombajiras, masters and mistresses who also appear in Umbanda ceremonies—such as Ritinha, Luziara, and Maria Padilha—raises a difficult question: after all, is Jurema Sagrada a branch of Umbanda or a separate, autonomous religion? To what extent does it incorporate Orixás from Candomblé or Xangô? This question persisted through many visits to Jurema houses and terreiros, both in the Northeast and elsewhere—for example, in Belo Horizonte (state of Minas Gerais) and Santo André (São Paulo)—without ever being fully resolved. On the contrary, this ambiguity, this indeterminacy of boundaries, seems to reveal something essential about this peculiar northeastern complex of Amerindian-African religious heritage.

Anthropologist Sandro Guimarães de Salles reports that Zefa de Tiíno, also known as Mestra Jardecilha, was a representative and inspector in Alhandra for the Federation of African Cults of the State of Paraíba,[5] an organization that sheltered and rescued Jurema from police persecution. The temple houses ilus, drums used for rhythms of clear African inspiration, which are absent from indigenous rituals where maracás predominate. Nina, Jardecilha's daughter, recounts that the matriarch received Exu. Her own son, Lucas, is a Candomblé priest, although he practices the rituals separately and presents himself only as Lucas Juremeiro. He acknowledges that "miscegenation" led to a loss of Jurema's identity—he cites the case of sementação (the implantation of a jurema-preta seed under the initiate's skin), which was not practiced by indigenous peoples or in Catimbó and was eventually assimilated under the influence of Candomblé. Indeed, it is common to hear from practitioners—such as Pai Ciriaco, Dona Raquel, and Nayanne in Alhandra, or Alexandre L'Omi L'Odó in Recife—that a juremeiro is born ready, requiring no initiatory or seclusion rites, although others advocate the necessity of baptism, sementação, and tombo.

In the specific case of Umbanda, the argument against the notion that Jurema Sagrada is a branch of it is based on anachronism: the indigenous and northeastern roots of Catimbó, from which it originated, are lost in the mists of colonial and pre-colonial times. As Alexandre states, "the time of Jurema's existence in the Northeast is infinitely greater than the time of Umbanda's existence in the country."[6] Umbanda emerged at the beginning of the twentieth century, according to what Luiz Antonio Simas calls its origin myth: on November 15, 1908, at the Spiritist Federation of Niterói (state of Rio de Janeiro), the young Zélio Fernandino de Moraes was taken to a session that was upended by the incorporation of a spirit who introduced himself as Caboclo das Sete Encruzilhadas. In a previous incarnation, the Caboclo was said to have been a Jesuit priest, Gabriel Malagrida, who was executed at the stake by the Holy Office in the nineteenth century. After this, Zélio would found the Templo Espírita Nossa Senhora da Piedade, which presented itself as Umbandist, Christian, and Brazilian.[7]

The mention of the crossroads ("encruzilhada"), caboclos (indigenous spirits), pretos velhos (African ancestors), and other elements of the newly emerged cult points, as Simas notes, to an obvious assimilation of African and Amerindian elements in a blend that, paradoxically, can also be seen as a process of whitening, through the imposition of Kardecist evolutionary discipline on a host of supposedly primitive entities lacking doctrine. This amalgam became institutionalized in the form of Umbanda state federations, which proliferated from 1939 onward, with the first appearing in Rio de Janeiro.[8] The Paraíba federation would be founded in 1966, when it began to register and protect Jurema terreiros that predated it. In this sense, at least in its institutionalized form, it is clear that Umbanda could not have been the source of Jurema Sagrada.

Quite another matter are elements of Jurema originating from the rich African matrix that some refer to generically as "macumbas," predating Umbanda. From very early on, well before urban syncretism—perhaps as early as the eighteenth century and certainly by the 19th—there were many exchanges between indigenous peoples and enslaved Africans, whether in settlements and adjacent plantations run by priests who owned slaves, or in camps—mocambos and quilombos—founded by those who escaped European domination, as well as in the cattle ranches of the backlands with their Black cowboys. From the santidades of the sixteenth century to the Candomblé de Caboclo of the 19th, there is a continuous thread which intertwines the use of jurema, pipes, and maracás with herbs, trances, and ancestor worship (eguns) common in African rites, as noted by Clélia Moreira Pinto.[9]

Mário de Andrade would say, among thousands of notes and records reproduced in the volume *Música de Feitiçaria no Brasil* (posthumously organized by Oneyda Alvarenga), that the Indigenous origin of Catimbó seemed to him indisputable, "the most intimately national aspect of our religiosity." There was contact with macumba, no doubt, the writer affirms, but the core of Catimbó mythology is Amazonian, the liturgy is largely Amerindian, and the music in general acquires a Lusitanian quality emptied of Portugal, with almost no trace of Africa (except in distinctly African elements dedicated to Afro-Brazilian Masters), According to him, it has a languor that evokes a Tapuia existence, a fusion of Portuguese and Amerindians.[10]

By emphasizing the Indigenous and European components of Catimbó, Mário de Andrade follows the notions of Câmara Cascudo, who hosted the São Paulo folklorist during his trip to Natal in 1928, when Andrade underwent a body-closing ritual in a terreiro. Cascudo, a pioneer in the study of religiosity that would give rise to today's Sacred Jurema, defines Catimbó as the result of a welcoming syncretism among the "Masters from Beyond," Africans, Indigenous peoples, and national mestizos,[11] like veins of the same block of marble, or three inseparable streams flowing to the sea. However, as he highlights the soothing services that Catimbó provides to the poor population of the Northeast, he privileges the European ingredients of the magical practices surrounding the jurema plant: "The processes of witchcraft, catimbó, and sorcery in Brazil are more than eighty percent of European origin." More than that, Catimbó practitioners would be responding to a universal human need, albeit a universality tinged with Eurocentrism, as can be seen when Cascudo summarizes the purpose of his book on Catimbó: "*Meleagro* seeks to highlight the antiquity of many of the seductive elements in catimbó," he writes.

> Antiquity of Greece and Rome, ancient Eastern traditions, secrets of the Middle Ages, would not weigh so heavily if they were not a continuity, a dark and stubborn river flowing into the freshest waters of the most modern achievements. The witches of Catimbó live in every country in the world. (Author's translation with the help of artificial intelligence)

Mestre and mestra are the titles reserved for great Catimbó and Jurema practitioners who, in life, demonstrate the ability to perform remarkable healings, give accurate advice, and cast or break powerful spells. After death, they become enchanted as entities who retain their titles, such as Mestra Jardecilha, Mestre Carlos, and Mestre Manoel Cadete. When they descend in Jurema Sagrada rituals, it is once again to work—that is, to perform healings, prescribe obligations, and deliver "messages," like those I received from Zé Pelintra, Zé Bebim, Malunguinho, and Cigana, or health remedies. Although pipe smoke is widely used—a practice of evident Amerindian origin—Cascudo associates this medicine of the poor for the poor less with shamans and African sorcerers than with healers and witches inheriting European magic, possessors of that other "science."

Upon becoming enchanted, mestras and mestres come to inhabit another plane of reality, in specific cities, states, or kingdoms. This mythological geography of Jurema also appears to have a clear European origin, as such administrative divisions, so to speak, would make little sense among Brazilian Indigenous peoples and enslaved Africans. The strong white contribution to Catimbó is also evident in the omnipresence of popular Catholicism of Iberian origin, further reinforced by Kardecist Spiritism from the nineteenth century on, with the advent of Umbanda.

This form of whitening of Afro-Amerindian Catimbó, which Cascudo in his more generous passages defines as the result of a welcoming syncretism, appears as degeneration among later generations of religion scholars, such as Roger Bastide, who sees Jurema practitioners as poor country folk condemned to a mediocre existence and attracted by the "pride of speaking with the enchanted"[12]: according to him, two entirely different collective psychologies are marked in Candomblé and Catimbó, that of the African and that of the Indigenous. But while the mythology of Candomblé is rich and complex, that of Catimbó would, in his opinion, be poor and incipient, because the ancient Indigenous mythology was lost in the disintegration of the original peoples, in the transition from local culture to the culture of the whites, who were willing to accept the rites but not the pagan dogmas, in their fidelity to Catholicism. For Bastide, Catimbó was conceived more as magic than as a true religion, due to its dangerous and fearsome elements and the persecutions by the Church and the police.

The fascination exerted on academics by the supposed African purity in Candomblé overshadowed the study of Catimbó for decades, following the pioneering works of Cascudo and Andrade in the first half of the nineteenth century, which would only be resumed in earnest from the 1970s onward, especially by authors from the Northeast such as René Vandezande. Although still little recognized in universities in the Southeast, a school of anthropological studies on Catimbó and Jurema Sagrada emerged in the 1990s with the work of Rodrigo de Azeredo Grünewald, who researched Indigenous jurema practices among the Atikum of Serra do Umã (Pernambuco); and Luiz Assunção and Sandro Guimarães de Salles, who focused on contemporary relations between Jurema and Umbanda, as can be seen from the titles of their books, respectively *O Reino dos Mestres: A tradição da Jurema na Umbanda nordestina* (the kingdom of the masters: the tradition of Jurema in Northeastern Umbanda, 2006) and *À Sombra da Jurema Encantada: Mestres juremeiros na Umbanda de Alhandra* (in the shadow of the enchanted Jurema: Jurema masters in the Umbanda of Alhandra, 2010). The trio would give rise to a series of master's dissertations and doctoral theses on Jurema, some of which are included in the bibliography of this book.

Assunção recounts that, when he began his ethnographic investigation, he was only familiar with Candomblé and Umbanda. For two years, he traveled through the interior of Paraíba, Pernambuco, Piauí, and Ceará states, when he discovered something more in the Umbanda terreiros—Jurema Sagrada. "It was what kept the house standing, what moved it," he said in an interview in May 2022, referring to the consultations given by the juremeiros, who are deeply knowledgeable about herbs, an Indigenous heritage: "One of the points I defend, the main one I wanted to show and went to seek in the backlands, was precisely that Jurema has always existed as a ritual practice." Intolerance caused it to become closed-off, he says, but Jurema has also always been, in this transition to the urban environment, a practice of small groups, centered around a living master in their community, who served the people of the group.

This is the process that Alexandre L'Omi L'Odó would later call "alvenarização,"[13] a neologism equivalent to "masonrization," when rituals originally practiced in the forest migrate to the rooms and kitchens of small brick houses to escape religious and police persecution. From the 1960s onward, institutionalized Umbanda allowed Jurema to leave the cramped spaces between four walls and spread to terreiros registered as Umbanda by practicing juremeiros. They play for Exu at the opening of rituals and then for the Jurema masters, summarizes Assunção. This is yet another form of invisibilization, parallel to the academic disregard for a religiosity seen as a degeneration of Candomblé or as an appendix to Umbanda, or at least as a concealment of the deeper roots of Jurema in the Amerindian-African past of the Northeast.

This would begin to change at the turn of the twenty-first century, when the identity movement led by figures such as Alexandre L'Omi L'Odó began to claim the precedence of Jurema Sagrada in the Northeast, focusing more on the backlands, where the balck jurema and the mixture of Black, Indigenous, and European populations thrive, than on the coast and the sugarcane-covered Zona da Mata shaped by enslaved labor, where some preferred to focus on the idealized African purity of Candomblé. In 2010, a census of terreiros conducted by the Ministry of Social Development and UNESCO in four Brazilian metropolitan regions (Belém, Belo Horizonte, Porto Alegre, and Recife) showed that Umbanda is the most practiced in the first three, but not in the Pernambuco metropolis, where 896 houses indicated Jurema as predominant, followed by Candomblé (703) and Umbanda (365).[14]

The neglect of Jurema by religion scholars from outside the Northeast still has effects today. The historian and anthropologist from Minas Gerais, Dilaine Soares Sampaio, already had a decade of studies on Afro-Brazilian religions when she was hired by the Federal University of Paraíba (UFPB), but she was unfamiliar with Jurema Sagrada. "Here, I freaked out, thinking I didn't know anything anymore," she said in a December 2022 interview. "I had to study. I felt the need to map the subject, which was much neglected. Bastide has only a single text on it." Her greatest surprise was coming across the work of Mário de Andrade. She would soon discover the works of Luiz Assunção and Sandro de Salles.

Sampaio was raised in Juiz de Fora (Minas Gerais), under the strict precepts of the Methodist Church, but the African matrix was not far from her family circle: an aunt was a daughter of Iemanjá; another older uncle, nicknamed "Vô," was a healer and had his own Caboclo and Preto Velho. After graduating in history from the Federal University of Juiz de Fora (UFJF), she began her scientific initiation with the anthropologist Fátima Tavares from Rio de Janeiro, being tasked with surveying the opinion of professional medical organizations regarding alternative practices in terreiros, which were to be visited by a colleague. However, he asked to switch roles, and the world opened up for her: on her first visit to the Candomblé house of Pai Angelo, she was deeply moved. She had planned to research the neopentecostalist Universal Church of the Kingdom of God for her master's, but her professor convinced her to study the Catholic discourse on Umbanda in the years 1940–65. For her doctorate, she conducted ethnography of the Casa Branca do Engenho Velho terreiro, of Mãe Stella de Oxóssi, in the state of Bahia.

In João Pessoa, Paraíba, where she moved in 2010 while still writing her doctoral dissertation on Candomblé, Sampaio encountered in the terreiros a blend of Umbanda, Nagô, and Jurema: "One day, I heard a pombajira song, but the embodiment was very different—the person possessed was not a pombajira, but a Jurema master, wearing a cangaceira hat" (a reference to the leather hat typical of the Northeast). The differences, however, ran much deeper than the mere characterization of the entities, reaching the level of what the researcher prefers to call cosmoperception—the matrix of notions that organizes the lived world, but is received through all the senses, with the body, without privileging vision and reason.

There are many elements specific to Jurema Sagrada: the pipe and smoke, black jurema as a power plant, maracás, cities where the enchanted beings dwell. It is true that in the oldest texts about Catimbó there is no mention of exus and pombajiras, nor of seclusion and initiation, but no religion remains static, Sampaio argues; rather, it continually reinvents tradition. Over these twelve years, she says, she has been able to see and understand Catimbó-Jurema better: "Is there a process of candomblization in some terreiros? Yes. Is there a strong influence from Umbanda? Yes. But Jurema is a religion distinct from Umbanda and Candomblé. I disagree, I do not see it as Northeastern Umbanda."

At a Masters' Festival attended by the specialist, there was a draft beer tower from which jurema wine flowed freely, and anyone could help themselves, though without experiencing any psychedelic effect. "I drank four gourds and cured my cold." The anthropologist prefers to speak of an expansion of consciousness, even if without the visual manifestations typical of ayahuasca visions. "The Master arrives, asks for a pipe and jurema wine. He comes down to work, to help people. He gives you the drink, but it is no longer just jurema—it can be beer, wine—it is sacralized," she explains. She does not consider herself a practitioner of Jurema, Umbanda, or Candomblé, but neither did she emerge unscathed, as a researcher, from frequenting the terreiros: "The field crosses into your personal life. There is no such thing as separating the researcher from the person you are. The entities mix everything, they don't care. They are there to do their work, and we are there to do ours."

Perhaps it is not even appropriate to designate this vortex of traditions, sacraments, and rituals that make up Jurema Sagrada by the term "syncretism," even in the generous sense given by Cascudo, who characterized it as welcoming syncretism. René Vandezande's proposal seems apt: to recover the concept of "bricolage" as applied to mythical thought by Claude Lévi-Strauss, in which heterogeneous elements, fragments, and remnants from the history of individuals and societies, are recreated as symbols within a new structure—not as categories in a classificatory system or as pieces shaped by a predetermined plan. Each catimbozeiro mobilizes the available elements in their own way, Vandezande teaches: "These symbols are mixed, related anew, and used again in ever new and original combinations. Without any reference, however, to the reality originally symbolized."

This is why the expectation of establishing what the doctrine of Jurema Sagrada is, and assigning it a defined place within the spectrum of Amerindian-African matrix religions in Brazil, proves so fruitless, not to say frustrating. The juremeiros themselves are often at odds with one another, each pontificating about what the true Jurema is—whether it involves sementação or not, whether exus and pombajiras have a place in it or not, whether jurema wine contains cachaça or not, whether only floral chintz shirts should be worn or if brightly colored satin ones are also acceptable, whether the songs should be accompanied only by maracás or if the ilu drum is also allowed, or which is the most correct list of enchanted cities and kingdoms.

As in trance, Jurema is the domain par excellence of freedom and creativity—that is, of a plasticity that resists all classification, of a carnivalization in which Eros and Dionysus reign, exus and pombajiras in the company of Kings Malunguinho and Canindé, of Cigana and Mestra Luziara, of Caboclos Pena Branca and Pena Preta, Pretas and Pretos Velhos, Cowboys, Sailors… The recent movement to revalue Jurema over the past three decades also implies a certain distancing from Umbanda and Candomblé, with their respective aspirations to institutionalization and purity. It is as if Kings Canindé and Malunguinho were claiming the right to enchanted citizenship so that their shamans and sorcerers can practice the eclectic magic of their ancestors without having to fear police and religious violence, academic disdain for supposed degeneration, or the moral repugnance aroused among whites by the mixture of macumbas and pajelanças with popular Catholicism and low spiritism, as it was pejoratively called in the first half of the twentieth century, when juremeiros were beaten by the police and taken into custody with their ritual tables on their heads, only to be forced to repeat their ritual at the police station.[15]

Much of the persecution once directed at Catimbó and now at Jurema is associated with witchcraft and sorcery, which the juremeiros themselves call left-hand works—that is, what the master provides to the client to protect them from harm or to inflict it on their enemies. It is a "symbolic garbage can," notes Alexandre L'Omi L'Odó, ready to receive everything that is cast out by society: "[…] Jurema, with the Science of the Left, would assume the ideology and identity of everything that has been rejected, excluded, vilified, and subjected to prejudice and violence in society." In his view, we cannot observe Jurema and reduce it solely to a religious experience seen through the lens of the Western logic of the sacred, which values its own hegemony, viewing the world from the perspective of Christianity and its notion of good within that cultural universe, which is very strong in Brazil.

The Left of Jurema would represent a break with the Judeo-Christian worldview, with its morality, ethics, and good customs. Because of this distinctive feature, it is subject to prejudice even from practitioners of Xangô or Candomblé.[16]

In contrast to the distant and silent Orixás, tricksters such as Malunguinho and Zé Pelintra are destined to be devalued by academic researchers, with their essentialist and fixist obsessions anchored in a Eurocentrism that dismisses as magic everything that differs from established religions with solid doctrines. Since the earliest scholars of Catimbó, such as Luís da Câmara Cascudo and Mário de Andrade, this disqualifying bias has been evident, as in the latter folklorist's description of Malunguinho after his visit to the terreiros of Natal (RN) accompanied by the former:

Malevolent African black sorcerer. Only practices evil. Works with his head on the ground. Works at midnight, with black cloths. Is capable of drinking more than one bottle of cauim [*jurema wine, possibly?*] at once, even two. No other spirit can undo his work. He is a backward spirit, dwells in lower worlds, and is generally not summoned. Orders the burial of cururu toads at the door of those who one wishes to harm. (Author's translation with the help of artificial intelligence)[17]

Caboclo Aboiador and Walter Benjamin in the Circle of Pankararé Praiás

Breakfast in the communal kitchen of the terreiro had just been enriched by the addition of fried tripe when the whistles sounded. Fifes announced the arrival of the delegation from Brejo do Burgo. Fireworks began to burst, and everyone left their food to head to the gateway of the sacred area of the Pankararé.[18] Thus began the Amaro Science Festival, open to the public since 1995. Leading the group from the village, fourteen kilometers away, was Edézia Maria da Conceição Feitoza, the Mãe Véia (Old Mother) of the terreiro, also known as Dona Deza, married to Chief Afonso Enéas.

The leader was welcomed by members of this Indigenous people of Bahia at the blue gates under a whitewashed masonry arch, topped with a cross, inscribed with "God bless everyone." Many of them, dressed in ceremonial caroá-fiber skirts, were organized in two lines starting from the entrance decorated with palm leaves. The whistling of the fifes, an instrument halfway between a whistle and a flute, gave way to the enveloping rattle of the maracás, always accompanying the toantes, songs of a few verses led by one person and repeated by all the others. An example:

In my science there are many enchanted beings to play
With the power of Jurema and the power of Juremá
In Amaro's terreiro we will celebrate
With the Enchanted Ones of the forests and my jatobá tree.

This is not just any jatobá, but the sacred tree that gave rise to Amaro's terreiro and serves as the dwelling of Caboclo Aboiador, an enchanted being who holds a central place in the Pankararé pantheon. Amid the scorched caatinga, a semi-arid biome, the ever-green canopy of the jatobá covers an enclosed area of ca. 400 m^2, which can only be entered through the circular structure called the Poró dos Homens. Only males over the age of 16 are allowed inside. There, the young men who will dance at night, dressed as praiás—characterized by garments also made of caroá, covering them from head to toe and representing the enchanted forces of the forest—gather. Under a small shelter is kept the jurema wine, the Pankararé sacrament to facilitate communication with the enchanted beings. "Jurema is what Our Lord blessed for the people to drink," the chief replied vaguely, after a few seconds of silence, when asked about the role of the beverage in the ritual. He limited himself to explaining that the wine can only be made with jurema-de-caboclo, a thornless variety of the Mimosa tree.

The Pankararé, like other Indigenous peoples of the Northeast, are very different from their Amazonian relatives, as they do not correspond to the stereotype of straight hair, almond-shaped eyes, and feather adornments (although at festivities such as Amaro's, headdresses are visible, some made of straw). This is a caboclo, mixed-race population whose customs were almost entirely erased during the colonial period, as happened to all other ethnic groups subjected to the forced settlements of the Jesuits and other Catholic orders. Invisibility also became a survival strategy, which is still evident today in the secrecy surrounding the so-called science, hence Afonso Enéas's reluctance to detail the preparation of jurema wine.

"I was heavily persecuted," the chief recounted in the interview on October 28, 2023. His bean and corn fields were burned, and his fences torn down. The conflicts involved squatters and even members of his own people who did not want to be identified as Indigenous when the federal government's Funai began the process of demarcating the territory in the 1980s. Today, a total of 47,500 hectares (475 km^2) have been officially recognized for the 2,400 Pankararé. The territory is located in the municipality of Glória (Bahia), near Paulo Afonso, on the right bank of the São Francisco River. With the construction of the Itaparica hydroelectric plant, many people were removed from their lands and relocated, including into the Indigenous area. A similar process accompanied the creation of the neighboring Raso da Catarina Ecological Station, a refuge for the endangered Lear's macaw. The region also became famous for the wanderings of Lampião's band, who camped in the area.

In 1979, during the struggle for demarcation, then-chief Ângelo Pereira Xavier was assassinated in an ambush, as reported by Elaine Patrícia de Sousa Oliveira, daughter-in-law of Dona Deza and Afonso Enéas, in her master's thesis.[19] Years later, Afonso would assume leadership and complete the process of recognition of the Pankararé territory. The conflicts persisted, making it difficult to carry out rituals that survived only in oral form, such as the toantes sung by Mãe Véia dos Praiás, Dona Deza, since her childhood.

While walking through the caatinga with the cattle, raised extensively in the fundo de pasto commons system,[20] Afonso one day was overcome by the scorching sun when the herd scattered. He found shade under a jatobá tree, the only vegetation with leaves in the endless dryness, and stopped to rest with his head against the trunk. He fell asleep. The cattle returned on their own and began licking his feet. There, the chief experienced the first apparition of Caboclo Aboiador, an enchanted entity at the heart of the Festa do Amaro, which his people began to organize at that very spot every last Saturday of October. "All the strength we had [in the struggle for demarcation] came from here, from Amaro," says the chief.

On the chapel altar, the bricolage of sertão religiosity is fully revealed. There are many images: besides Caboclo Aboiador, an Indigenous man with a bare torso and leather hat, there are statuettes of Padre Cícero, Jesus Christ, Saint George, Iemanjá, Caboclo Pena Branca, Our Lady of Aparecida, Cosmas and Damian… After the arrival of the procession led by Dona Deza and the ensuing toré, the next ritual of the Festa do Amaro is the chief's blessings in the chapel. He leads a toante with verses such as:

I am with God
With God I am
I am Caboclo Aboiador
Protect this house where we are
Protect those who have arrived and are here

Afterward, the midday prayer takes place in the small church. In the crowded space, toantes and the prayers of a complete rosary follow one another, sung under the guidance of three elders. There are incorporations of enchanted beings, such as the Capitão received by Dona Deza, an entity whose proper name cannot be revealed by the Pankararé. As everyone was leaving the little temple, I approached Mãe Véia to thank her for her people's hospitality. The lady embraced me with strong arms and began to utter blessings, asking for the mantle of Our Lady to cover me with love. I broke down in tears on that woman's shoulder, not understanding why. It was both unsettling and overwhelming, an emotion that returns every time I revisit the moment. It takes a lot of faith to remain an atheist, a friend jokes. Patrícia, Dona Deza's daughter-in-law, explains that in reality I was embraced by the Capitão, not by the Amaro matriarch.

A little before the midday prayer, in the enclosure of the Poró dos Homens under the jatobá tree, a man was serving jurema wine. I joined the line, knelt, and drank a gourdful of the liquid prepared cold, only with water and fibers from the mashed jurema root, as Chief Afonso had explained (other recipes may include honey, spices, fruits, and cachaça). There was no noticeable psychedelic effect. For the Indigenous peoples of the Northeast, experiencing contact with the enchanted beings does not depend on that. Communion with the spirits of nature arises from the ritual as a whole: torés, maracás, toantes, smoke from the campiôs (conical pipes), caroá costumes, prayers, penances, praiás, the imposing canopy of the jatobá tree, the celebration of cultural roots, and the sharing of meals freely offered by the festival organizers, with plenty of meat, couscous, rice, and beans. Enchantment was clearly visible on everyone's faces, with no shortage of smiles. The children, in particular, seemed filled with a proud enthusiasm as they wore their caroá skirts and maracás tucked into their aiós (fiber bags).

In the late afternoon, a long procession took place through the caatinga. Leading the cortege was a platform bearing the image of Caboclo Aboiador, surrounded by other figures such as Our Lady, Saint Barbara, and Cosmas and Damian, and carried by pairs who took turns, including women like Patrícia. The procession's destination was the cross on the hill ahead, dedicated to Maria Mulambeira, another prominent entity in the Pankararé pantheon. The walk over the scorching soft sand allowed for only a few stops at certain trees, such as umbuzeiros, which were honored by the Indigenous participants tying colored ribbons to them. Beneath the whitewashed cross, where the words "Maria and José" were written in blue, Chief Afonso sat beside the platform. Standing next to him, Patrícia raised the maracá to accompany the toantes and prayers, visibly ecstatic. Several people sought niches among the rocks to light candles and shelter them from the wind sweeping across the caatinga.

The return descent to Amaro's yard took a different, shorter, and steeper path. The entire route, in the Indigenous perspective, resembles the traditional oval representation of the Catholic rosary. The sun set during the walk back, tinting the white forest—a tangle of leafless trunks and branches—with reddish hues. On the opposite side of the sunset, the full moon rose, but with a missing slice on its right flank—a partial lunar eclipse, to complete the scene.

Upon arrival at the festival grounds, a group of apprentice praiás boys emerged from the Children's Poró for their performance. They danced and sang in the twilight, warmly applauded for their efforts to continue the tradition. The true praiás would appear only after dinner. Once again, the sound of whistles was heard, coming from the forest to the left of the jatobá and the Men's Poró. Two dozen ghostly figures descended, filling the yard, illuminated only by moonlight and bonfires. With their "folguedo" (costume) concealing their feet, their quick steps made them seem to glide over the sand. The mask, with two small holes for the eyes, is topped by a circular feather ornament, making the figures appear even taller and more imposing. Colorful capes on their backs bore white crosses, reminiscent of medieval crusaders.

A row of women, with Dona Deza at the center, led the toantes for the praiás to dance. After a few evolutions in line, some accompanied by women, they gathered in circles and let out cries—half growls—producing in unison a visceral sound—*Huh! Huh!*—that resonated in the chest of everyone present. It was the highlight of the festival. Dozens, perhaps hundreds, of fireworks were set off throughout the celebration and into the night. A toré followed, with everyone participating.

The blending of the three streams of Catimbó-Jurema—Amerindian, African, and European—presents a tough nut for the classificatory machinery of Western science. At first, an author like Cascudo chose to emphasize the waters of Iberian witchcraft as dominant, which he considers a universal constant in the human species, to the point of choosing as the enigmatic title of his pioneering book the name of a prince from Greek mythology (Meleager) who dies when his mother, enraged that he killed her brothers, throws into the fire the log to which the hero's life was bound: "Who killed Meleager was the Magic that lives in Catimbó."[21] Academic knowledge always tends to highlight a dominant, essential component, and the folklorist from Rio Grande do Norte opts for the colonizer, even if apparently less civilized. Name, organization, functioning, everything is obscure, mixed, confused, writes Câma Cascudo. It is a sum of influence and convergence, like all cults: "The most decisive feature is European witchcraft, the 'master' and his prestige, the consultation without the obligation of adherence."[22]

Recently, after a hiatus in academic production on Jurema, some have preferred to emphasize Umbanda, such as Luiz Assunção and Sandro de Salles, while others highlight the Amerindian roots and their resurgence in today's Northeast, such as Rodrigo Grünewald, Alexandre L'Omi L'Odó, and Miguel Bittencourt. Roberto Motta even organized the process of cultural accumulation in Catimbó into three stages, according to Grünewald and Savoldi. The first would be linked to the introduction of the figure of the master and magical techniques of European origin, as Cascudo emphasizes. The second would correspond to the influence of Kardecist Spiritism, which, even before the creation of Umbanda, codified a popular mediumship. The last would refer to the influence of "Afro-Carioca" religions, such as the introduction of new spirits (like the exus) or animal sacrifice—elements previously unknown to the juremeiros.[23]

Everyone, however, recognizes and emphasizes the indelibly mixed nature of this religion. Jurema Sagrada is not Umbanda, except when it is.

Its inherent plasticity has also served the role it has played—and continues to play—in the cultural survival of marginalized populations and peoples, such as the Pankararé of Brejo do Burgo (Bahia), the Fulni-ô of Águas Belas (Pernambuco), or the Potiguara of Baía da Traição (Paraíba). A kind of serial syncretism, bricolage, or foundational eclecticism has led to a situation in which today, Indigenous peoples of the backlands—where the roots of Catimbó that flourished in the forest zone are found—receive back from the coast the fruits of Umbandization in the second half of the twentieth century and sing points, toantes, and lines about Zé Pelintra, Exu, Pombajira, and Cowboys—such as the Caboclo Aboiador venerated at the Amaro Science Festival. In their own way,[24] caboclos perform, through the power of Jurema, the miracle of continuity amid the devastating trajectory of the Northeast and all of Brazil, like the angel of history, the one who looks backward and would like to stay, awaken the dead, and make whole what has been smashed, as Walter Benjamin wrote in his *Theses on the Philosophy of History*.

Notes

1. Some Jurema Sagrada houses practice initiation rituals such as the tombo (special ceremonies with offerings to a person's guides) and sementação (implantation of black jurema seeds under the skin).
2. Marcus Vinícius Rios Barreto, *Malunguinho: Da narrativa histórica à estética digital*. São Paulo: USP, 2021. Doctoral thesis. p. 52.
3. Alexandre L'Omi L'Odó, *Malunguinho: Pressupostos juremológicos para sua compreensão da Jurema Sagrada*. Olinda: Casa das Matas do Reis Malunguinho and Quilombo Cultural Malunguinho, 2022. p. 6.
4. Available at: <https://youtu.be/rOndYeYcIX4?si=V-hwIa1iwUhbFJJk> . Accessed: Dec. 20, 2024.
5. Sandro Guimarães de Salles, *À Sombra da Jurema Encantada*. Recife: Editora UFPE, 2010. p. 93.
6. Alexandre L'Omi L'Odó, *Juremologia: Uma busca etnográfica para sistematização de princípios da cosmovisãoda Jurema Sagrada*. Recife: Universidade Católica de Pernambuco, 2017. Master's thesis in Social Sciences. p. 138.
7. Luiz Antonio Simas, *Umbandas: Uma história do Brasil*. Rio de Janeiro: Civilização Brasileira, 2023. pp. 97–8.
8. Sandro Guimarães de Salles, *À Sombra da Jurema Encantada*, p. 86.
9. Clélia Moreira Pinto, *Saravá Jurema Sagrada*. Recife: UFPE, 1995. pp. 36; 42–4.
10. Mário de Andrade, *Música de Feitiçaria no Brasil*. São Paulo: Livraria Martins Editora, 1963. p. 266 (notes 1152 and 1153).
11. Luís da Câmara Cascudo, *Meleagro*. Rio de Janeiro: Agir, 1978. p. 16.

12. Roger Bastide, "Catimbó," in Reginaldo Prandi (Ed.), *Encantaria Brasileira*. Rio de Janeiro: Pallas, 2011. p. 154.
13. Alexandre L'Omi L'Odó, *Juremologia*, p. 27.
14. Ministério do Desenvolvimento Social e Combate à Fome, *Alimento: Direito sagrado—pesquisa socioeconômica e cultural de povos e comunidades tradicionais de terreiros*. Brasília, DF: MDS, Secretaria de Avaliação e Gestão da Informação, 2011. p. 138.
15. Francisco Sales de Lima Segundo, *Memória e Tradição da Ciência da Jurema em Alhandra (PB)*. João Pessoa: UFPB, 2015. Dissertation (Master's in Anthropology). pp. 60–1.
16. Alexandre L'Omi L'Odó, *Juremologia*, p. 171.
17. Mário de Andrade, *Música de Feitiçaria no Brasil*, pp. 114–5.
18. This account of the Amaro Science Festival was originally published on December 5, 2023 in *Folha de S.Paulo* under the title "Indígenas bebem vinho Sagrado para celebrar entidades da mata." Available at: <https://www1.folha.uol.com.br/ilustrissima/2023/12/indigenas-bebem-vinho-sagrado-para-celebrar-entidades-da-mata.shtml>. Accessed: Dec. 20, 2024.
19. Elaine Patrícia de Sousa Oliveira, *A Mulher na Ciência do Amaro*. Paulo Afonso: Universidade Estadual da Bahia, 2023. Dissertation (Master's). p. 19.
20. Common use areas, where animals roam freely.
21. Luís da Câmara Cascudo, *Meleagro*, p. 23.
22. [20] Ibid., p. 23.
23. Rodrigo Grünewald and Robson Savoldi, "Contexto e Usos da Jurema," in Beatriz Caiuby Labate and Sandra Lucia Goulart (Eds.), *O Uso de Plantas Psicoativas nas Américas*. Rio de Janeiro: Gramma/Neip, 2019. p. 330.
24. Estevão Palitot and Rodrigo Grünewald, "O País da Jurema: Revisitando as fontes históricas do ritual Atikum." *Acervo*, May-Aug. 2021. p. 5.

Juremahuasca, a Sacrament to Challenge All Doctrines

"Jurema is the cosmos in a little cup," Rodrigo Grünewald often repeats about the beverage and the plant that have shaped his career as an anthropologist. He adopted the phrase after hearing it in the late 1990s from an elderly man, in his eighties, Natanael, who attended one of the closed rituals Rodrigo organized at his retreat in Jacarepaguá, in the western part of Rio de Janeiro. In fact, it was *half* a cup: for safety, since it was the man's first experience with the entheogen, Rodrigo gave him only half the usual dose. After 30 minutes or so, the man exclaimed: "Get this away from me, take this power for yourself! No one can handle this power!" Hours later, once the effects had worn off, Natanael explained in his own way what he had experienced: "This jurema of yours is the cosmos in a little cup."[1]

However, this was not the so-called jurema wine of indigenous origin, whose ritual use the Rio de Janeiro anthropologist had been studying since 1990, when he traveled to Carnaubeira da Penha, in Pernambuco, for ethnographic work with the Atikum people, which would become the subject of his master's thesis.[2] Instead of *anjucá*, a reddish beverage (hence the description as wine) obtained from the cold infusion of macerated *Mimosa tenuiflora* root bark, the ceremonies in Jacarepaguá featured *juremahuasca*, a psychonautical innovation introduced in Brazil on January 6, 1997, Dia de Reis (Three Kings' Day, an important religious date in Brazil), by the natural therapist Wanda Maria da Silveira Barbosa, then recently arrived from the Netherlands and better known as Yatra, with Rodrigo as host.

The anthropologist had followed an unusual path before becoming a protagonist in the initial act that would spread the power of jurema throughout Brazil, far beyond the backlands and Northeastern coast where

© The Author(s), under exclusive license to Springer Nature Switzerland AG 2026
M. Leite, *The Psychedelic Science of the Jurema Tree*, Copernicus Books,
https://doi.org/10.1007/978-3-032-22705-8_5

it had been confined for centuries. The son of journalist, translator, and film critic José Lino Grünewald, he grew up surrounded by literature, cinema, agnosticism, and counterculture. In the 1980s, he "partied hard," like many others of the sex-drugs-and-rock'n'roll generation, and wanted nothing to do with religion.

As an undergraduate in social sciences at the Federal University of Rio de Janeiro (UFRJ), he was a student of Clarice Novaes da Mota, a social psychologist and ethnobotanist who pioneered the study of jurema among northeastern ethnic groups such as the Kariri-Xocó. Influenced by her, he was led to study the Atikum, defending his thesis in 1993, but spent only a few months in Serra do Umã, leaving due to escalating land conflicts in the region that opposed farmers and settlers to Indigenous groups such as the Atikum.

The turning point came in 1995, the year he met the sociologist of ayahuasca religions Edward John Baptista das Neves MacRae, who was introduced to him in João Pessoa during a congress of the Brazilian Association of Anthropology. Rodrigo proposed to MacRae a panel on religiosity surrounding jurema for the 1 st Meeting on Studies of Religious and Social Rituals and the Use of Psychoactive Plants, which would take place in Salvador in the second half of that year. His presentation at the panel caught the attention of the Colombian-born Santo Daime practitioner Luis Eduardo Luna, who asked him for a copy of the floppy disk, the digital storage medium in use at the time. That same year, Rodrigo was invited by his acquaintance Philippe Bandeira de Mello to a daime (ayahuasca) ritual at the Barquinha church, where he drank the Amazonian psychedelic tea for the first time. "I didn't believe in anything, but I felt a certain resignation—there is something more than myself," he recalls.[3] At these rituals he met Jonathan Ott, an American psychonaut who would play a decisive role in the dissemination of juremahuasca in Brazil and worldwide. Ott was in Rio for a congress of the ayahuasca church União do Vegetal (UDV) held at the Hotel Glória.

A brief aside on juremahuasca is warranted here. As the neologism suggests, the preparation is defined as an analogue of ayahuasca, or *anahuasca*. Black jurema contains in its roots a high concentration of the same psychedelic (DMT) found in chacruna, one of the two ingredients in the Amazonian brew, which also includes the mariri vine. Without the vine's inhibitors, DMT would not reach the brain or produce the visions characteristic of ayahuasca. Since Indigenous jurema wine generally lacks these inhibitors, it rarely produces noticeable psychedelic effects. To achieve this effect from

Mimosa tenuiflora, the technique emerged of adding seeds from an exotic plant, Syrian rue (*Peganum harmala*), to the preparation.

To this combination of black jurema with Syrian rue, Jonathan Ott gave the name *juremahuasca*. Rodrigo would only come to know and drink this ayahuasca analogue two years after the congress, following a triangulation of events with vertices in the Netherlands, Mexico, and Brazil.

The Path of Black Jurema: From the Netherlands and Mexico to Rio De Janeiro

The Brazilian daimista Wanda Maria da Silveira Barbosa adopted the religious name Yatra, which in Hindi means something like "pilgrimage." Based in Amsterdam, where she founded the organization Friends of the Forest, she dedicated herself there to treating drug addicts, particularly heroin users, with the help of ayahuasca. "Right in the first ritual I hit a wall," she recounted, laughing, during a live broadcast of the Rede Saberes Ancestrais e Cura Integrativa (SACI, acronym that in English means Network of Ancestral Knowledge and Integrative Healing) with Rodrigo Grünewald and the shaman Amanacy Potiguara, on June 29, 2022.[4] Heroin addicts wanted to quit the drug but rejected the Santo Daime doctrine, resistant to a ceremony with that group of people in garb ("fardados", in Portuguese, a reference to the formal white and navy-blue clothing worn in the Santo Daime church).

In addition to the reluctance of European addicts, Yatra reports that she began to face an additional challenge: obtaining the brew cooked with Amazonian plants and using it legally in the Netherlands. Seeking an alternative, in 1995 she contacted Jonathan Ott, the American chemist and psychonaut based in Veracruz, Mexico, who since 1976 had been publishing books and articles on hallucinogenic plants[5] and in 1992 released *Pharmacotheon*,[6] a classic of psychedelic literature in which he proposed the idea of *anahuasca*, which would dispense with chacruna and the mariri vine, sometimes referred to as *pharmahuasca*, combining other sources of DMT and inhibitors.

In 1996, Yatra began using juremahuasca following Ott's recipe, which included Syrian rue seeds, commercially available and used as a traditional medicine, as a spice, and also as a source of red pigment. The other ingredient was black jurema, initially *Mimosa tenuiflora* from Mexico, where the tree is called *tepezcohuite* and is used as an herbal remedy for wounds and burns. Yatra held sessions every three days, roughly the duration of the so-called *afterglow* left by the drink, to prevent participants from disconnecting from the positive sensations mediated by the beverage. She maintained the administration of methadone, though, an opioid substitute for heroin used in harm reduction, but mixed it with honey and water, gradually reducing the opioid concentration without the addicts' knowledge. After three weeks, when everyone was free from the terrible symptoms of withdrawal syndrome, which should have appeared after reducing the dose and then stopping methadone altogether, Yatra revealed the ruse. "You tricked us," the addicts protested. "I tricked you with the greatest love," the healer replied.

Yatra stated during the SACI network panel with Grünewald and Amanacy that she had been addicted to cocaine and heroin for many years and only overcame her dependence with daime. If the brew had freed her from addiction, she was convinced it would rescue them as well. The substitution of daime with juremahuasca proved even better than expected: "It was beautiful. I left the doctrine [Santo Daime], gave up the garb, received many hymns from Jurema, the Cabocla in my heart. It is an endless path: one comes to know oneself without judgment," the therapist said during the livestream. The addicts not only were non-believers, but had not even known spirituality, she claimed. "They were blind. They didn't even know what soul, cabocla, or spirit is. I didn't even try to explain: I just applied the teachings of Jurema."

They didn't know what to expect, she told the online audience. They just didn't want doctrine or uniforms. Jurema showed them what to do, turned on the light, so to say, and everything that was in the dark appeared, but in a gentle, genuine way: "This Cabocla is here to help. Something that simple: kindness to oneself. Jurema lifts that veil. We arrive thinking we have a somber destiny and leave with a new vision of life, of what love is."

Knowing that black jurema also grew in the semi-arid backlands of the Northeast and was used in Indigenous rituals, Yatra sought out Luis Eduardo Luna for information to organize an expedition to that region of her home country, Brazil. Luna then sent her the diskette with Grünewald's lecture from a year earlier in Salvador, along with the contact details of the anthropologist from Rio de Janeiro. It was with surprise that one day in late 1996, in front of the black computer screen, he received a message from Yatra in green letters, he recounts in the book *Jurema*, establishing contact so that he could serve as a bridge for her to meet jurema-using Indigenous communities.

Grünewald welcomed Yatra to Rio in January 1997. On Three Kings' Day, they organized a ceremony at the Jacarepaguá house with the juremahuasca she had brought from Europe, attended by Philippe Bandeira de Mello and other members of the Barquinha congregation. "There is a pre-Yatra moment and a post-Yatra moment," the anthropologist says of the Rio de Janeiro psychonautic scene in the 1990s, which, propelled by juremahuasca, began to break away from the orbit of the Santo Daime tradition and its doctrine, making room for more eclectic ceremonies, blending mantras, Umbanda chants, Sufi music, Jurema lines, and Santo Daime hymns to enrich the rituals and journeys. Anthropologists have a habit of creating boxes, the researcher notes, but Jurema transcended everything—Catimbó, Umbanda, and so on: "Is there not value generation in nature and the cosmos? It is human arrogance to think that only we humans create value. [...] The children of Jurema know what I mean. She communicates something that seems infinite."[7]

After the inaugural juremahuasca session in Rio, Yatra headed to the esoteric city of Alto Paraíso (state of Goiás), where she held juremahuasca circles with friends who were *sannyasins*, followers of the controversial Indian guru Rajneesh Chandra Mohan Jain (1931–1990), known as Osho. In 2000, she participated in the founding of the Mãe D'Água temple there, having temporarily moved to Brazil after being prevented from continuing her work with substance abuse patients in the Netherlands, where DMT had been banned. During her 1997 visit, from Alto Paraíso she traveled to Salvador, where she stayed at MacRae's house. He and other anthropologists accompanied her on visits to Indigenous villages in the backlands, such as the Atikum communities, staying at the home of chief Ana. Yatra brought with her Syrian rue seeds to make juremahuasca, which she introduced to the drinkers of the traditional jurema wine, as Grünewald recounts in his book. There, she learned about Atikum rituals and, on her own initiative, prepared jurema mixed with *Peganum harmala*—an experience that, when recalled by locals, is not described in a positive or significant way. They only mention the woman who arrived with friends, encouraging them to prepare jurema differently. The Atikum did not notice any difference between their jurema and the one served by Yatra, although in one account, a woman later remarked that when she went to sleep after working with Yatra's jurema, she felt "a little high."[8]

Yatra herself, however, recounted on the SACI network panel in 2022, with Rodrigo and Amanacy, that ten members of the Atikum people drank her juremahuasca and that her hostess's mother fell to the floor, "boom!" All the Indigenous people turned to the outsider "with those wide eyes," angrily, and she thought they would not let her leave. She sat beside the elderly woman, placed her hand on her head, and began to sing her hymns, asking Cabocla Jurema for help in that situation. "Suddenly she got up, started dancing the toré in the middle of the room, and said: 'Huh, was I at home?' What a relief," Yatra recalled during the livestream, laughing heartily.

Before returning to the Netherlands, Yatra was again in Rio, where she prepared juremahuasca in Jacarepaguá, teaching Grünewald and Bandeira de Mello how to make the drink with Syrian rue. The recipe also included flowers known as angel's trumpets (*Brugmansia suaveolens*), which contain powerful alkaloids such as scopolamine and atropine, capable of inducing delirium and stupor. The recipe included three decoctions, using a single flower for fifteen people, but in the preparations he would make in the following years, the anthropologist used angel's trumpet only twice: "The effect is dark, swampy. It lingers, heavy, not luminous like Rio [de Janeiro] and DMT." His juremahuasca ceremonies were home-based, restricted to a few friends and acquaintances. His path diverged significantly from that of his friend and fellow juremahuasca practitioner Bandeira de Mello, who in the same year founded the Holistic Circle Ark of the Blue Mountain, after six years leading a Barquinha branch in Rio that was dissolving, as its leader told Marcos Albuquerque. In 1997, he received jurema, learning its preparation in a quantity sufficient to work for a year, from Yatra's hands: in the absence of daime, jurema was the sacred plant that inaugurated and blessed the Ark, his new place of work.[9]

Grünewald, for his part, took other paths. He passed a civil service exam to become a tenured professor at the Federal University of Campina Grande (state of Paraíba) and even served as vice president of the Barquinha, responsible for a branch of the church in the city of Campina Grande. He drank daime or jurema wine every week, recited the Lord's Prayer in the rituals, and during a pilgrimage in honor of Our Lady, he once saw the passage of souls before him. As the agnostic he was, reason told him it was not possible, but his eyes filled with tears. "Man, just keep quiet and accept this thing," he told himself. He thought he should baptize, but did not want to take the Catholic Church's preparatory course—he ended up receiving the Christian sacrament from an Orthodox priest. Yet his religiosity continued to balance on the tension between reason and faith: "In the light [under the effect of DMT], I see a lot of things and I say: this is real, it's not a hallucination, it's not tryptamine," he said in a 2023 interview. "Soon after, I'm not seeing it anymore and, working [intellectually], in remembrance I think: how could I have thought that was real? [I was] suggestible and so on."

He continued to use daime, with the leaves and vine he grows at home, without resorting to Syrian rue or black jurema, but now rarely partakes: "I started to feel my mind was overloaded with information, so I cut back, and the thing cools off when you don't practice much, the flame of faith fading away, fading away." In the year before our conversation, he had drunk the tea at most three times. Part of this drift can be attributed to jurema, which, unlike daime, does not carry the weight of an institutionalized church and thus does not lead to the indoctrination that Yatra's Dutch addicts rejected. Ayahuasca and its doctrines were ultimately abandoned by Yatra herself, after she heard instructions from Cabocla Jurema to that effect. Grünewald, for his part, did not receive such a strong calling to continue working with others, much less to follow the path of institutionalization adopted by Bandeira de Mello:

> Such a powerful force of connection with the cosmos, all possibilities, the total subjunctive—not the imperative of faith, of belief, but the subjunctive that everything is possible. To offer such a strong drink... this is no joke. We become more responsible, or more fearful, or more tired. (Author's translation with the help of artificial intelligence)

The anthropologist maintains sporadic contact with the Atikum, no longer to record, classify, or categorize what they do. From the close coexistence in the past remains the memory of walking in the forest with them after drinking jurema wine and, even without any obvious psychedelic effect, being overtaken by a magical and collective feeling of communion with nature, opposed to the rational separation between the profane and the sacred that makes so little sense in Amerindian worldviews. The first thing is to break into a wide smile, he recalls: "It gives one a sense of fulfillment, in the sense of integration with nature. Experiencing nature as enchanted is, for me, the very rich characteristic of jurema." He also retained the conviction that the voice of nature is as legitimate as that of science, and that to be able to hear it one must remain silent, as taught to him by shaman Augusto after his persistent questioning about the meaning of the interesting iconography engraved on a campiô (Indigenous pipe): "Rodrigo, don't you know that everything good comes in silence?".

Rodrigo spoke little at the 2022 panel. In the opening, he recounted how Yatra introduced him to juremahuasca, a milestone in his life, and thanked her for the journey they shared in jurema and spirituality. After nearly two hours of debate, which he listened to in silence, he was called upon to give his final contribution and reflected on why jurema did not have the same impact and reach as daime in the countercultural scene of the 1970s and 80s, even though it was closer and more accessible in the Northeast than ayahuasca in the remote Amazon, near the border with Peru and Colombia. In his view, the backpackers who ventured into the forest were seeking a supposed Indigenous purity, a clear and original source from which they could drink an elixir that would enable them to find an alternative path to integration into a society corroded by the military dictatorship (1964–1985).

Jurema, on the other hand, offered the proverbial image of mestizaje, seen here and there as degradation, used as it was by Indigenous people who still preferred not to claim their Indigenous identity, amid bloody land conflicts, and who had not been able to preserve their original rituals and languages after centuries of forced resettlement and religious or police repression. The anthropologist concluded his remarks by noting that the strength of jurema, in fact, lies precisely in its ability to transcend the dubious myth of cultural purity, and he defended it by saying that we need to break this prejudice against a plant used by people who speak Portuguese, mestizo in soul, body, speech, and blood:

> People separate the sacred from the profane too much, as if the sacred were [only] there in the ritual. What we are doing here is just as sacred as when we are speaking with spirits in rituals. We need to end these dichotomies and bring the sacred back into our daily lives. (Author's translation with the help of artificial intelligence)

Yatra was the last to say goodbye on the panel, and did so with a few words: "Much peace, much light, much love." Suffering from a serious illness, imperceptible in the video where she appeared rosy-cheeked and laughing animatedly, almost a month later she decided to have the equipment that kept her alive turned off, so she could make the passage, as it is said in her circle. It was on July 25, a date said to have been chosen because it is the "day out of time" in the Mayan lunar calendar, the day that belongs neither to the past year nor to the coming year.

Trance and Transcendence for All with the Pharmacologists of the Underworld

Two *sui generis* researchers were fundamental in spreading the worldwide fame of DMT from ayahuasca and juremahuasca as accessible entheogens: Jonathan Ott, who introduced the latter brew in the Netherlands and, indirectly, in Brazil through Yatra; and Richard Strassman, author of the influential book DMT*: The Spirit Molecule*, published in 2000. Seven years earlier, Ott had published his entheogenic bible, *Pharmacotheon*, with 639 pages in the English edition and 735 in Spanish.

The prologue to this compendium of psychedelic drugs was written by none other than Albert Hofmann, the Sandoz laboratory chemist who synthesized LSD in 1938 in Switzerland and discovered its lysergic effect on the brain in 1943. Both achievements are recounted in his autobiographical book *LSD: Mein Sorgenkind*, which was translated into English by Ott himself and published in 1980 under the title LSD*: My Problem Child*. In the introduction, the Swiss chemist highlights the most remarkable feature of

Pharmacotheon: the fact that it is all based on self-experimentation. That is, the author did not rely solely on chemical analyses to describe each drug, but ingested or injected them himself in order to describe the subjective effects triggered by the substances—description known as phenomenology.

Ott himself recounted in a 1998 interview[10] that he took the manuscript, begun in 1979 or 1980, out of the drawer after reading another classic of psychedelic literature, *PiHKAL: A Chemical Love Story* by Ann and Alexander Shulgin, which narrates the couple's experiences with the psychoactive compounds "Sasha" produced in his home laboratory and consumed with his wife and a circle of psychonaut friends. In the interview, Ott reproaches himself for having given in to self-censorship, which he attributes to the prevailing conservative political climate in the United States—he would later exile himself to Mexico after the 1980 election of Ronald Reagan, the conservative Republican president who today would seem a statesman compared to Donald Trump. He settled in Veracruz and moved to a property he named Ololiuhqui, after a sacred plant traditionally used in Mexico whose seeds contain LSA, a close relative of LSD. In the prologue, Hofmann explains why he considers self-experimentation and phenomenology important; for him, Ott's mystical experiences with entheogens and with nature decisively shaped the American's worldview and life path: "He acknowledges how these drugs opened his eyes to the wonder of that deeper, all-encompassing reality, into which we are all born as a part of the creation." In his view, this reality, described by all the great mystics and founders of religions, is the true kingdom of heaven destined for humanity. "There is, however, a fundamental distinction; whether one knows of this reality only from the reports of others, or whether one has experienced it personally in beatific moments; spontaneously or with the aid of entheogenic drugs."[11]

Ott was born in New Haven, Connecticut, in the eastern United States. In the biographical note that opens the Spanish edition of *Pharmacotheon*, the Catalan Josep Maria Fericgla describes him as a typical *self-made man*, "creative, tenacious, suggestive, and free." To avoid being drafted for the Vietnam War, from 1968 on he spent three years traversing the underworld of American society, where he came into contact with LSD. He graduated in chemistry from the University of Washington in the Pacific Northwest, where in 1973 he attended a lecture by Richard Evans Schultes, another luminary in the psychedelic field, who published the illustrated volume *Plants of the Gods* in 1992, with Hofmann and Christian Rätsch as co-authors. Schultes invited Ott to visit his specialized library at Harvard University, according to Fericgla, which would happen the following year. At that meeting, Ott was introduced to Robert Gordon Wasson, another giant of psychedelia, the banker and mycologist who had brought the sacred mushrooms of the Mazatec people in Mexico to Western attention in a 1957 *Life* magazine article titled "Seeking the Magic Mushroom." Wasson, in turn, invited him to his own home in Danbury, Connecticut, a visit that changed Ott's destiny: he abandoned formal graduate studies to become an apprentice of Schultes, Wasson, and Hofmann, according to Fericgla. Two years later, his first book on ethnobotany would be published: *Hallucinogenic Plants of North America.*

In 1979, dissatisfied with the pejorative connotation attached to the term "psychedelic" in the prohibitionist wave of demonization of LSD sparked by the War on Drugs, Ott, together with Wasson, Carl Ruck, Jeremy Bigwood, and Danny Staples, proposed the neologism *entheogen,* derived from Greek roots encapsulating the notion of "generating the divine within," to designate drugs that induce ecstasy and have traditionally been used as shamanic or religious inebriants, as well as their active principles and synthetic analogues. Ott developed a conception of entheogens that was at once mystical and naturalistic, viewing them as a universal resource for contacting the divine— an impulse he believed to be present even in other animal species, not just humans. In this quest, there would be no fundamental difference between explorers of the past and those of the future:

> May the shaman and the scientist now join hands and work together … may the psychonaut henceforth be accepted and cherished as a brave explorer of the great unknown, beyond yet somehow within, as vast and uncharted (and fraught with peril) as the trackless voids of interstellar space!

Graced by other sacred visions, his life was transformed and enriched: "I have become an initiate to the sacred Mysteries of antiquity, what the ancient Greeks called an *epoptes,* one who has seen the holy."

Such ecstasy would correspond to experiencing the universe less as matter than as energy—a vague and undefined concept (certainly not the physical definition) that would henceforth spread throughout the psychedelic and New Age esoteric milieu. In Western culture, however, the cosmos appears only as matter, eradicating the possibility of ecstasy and the understanding that every place is sacred, Ott argues, which would lend entheogens a missionary, proto-environmentalist virtue—an association that indeed permeated and defined the entire counterculture: "" I firmly believe that contemporary spiritual use of entheogenic drugs is one of humankind's brightest hopes for overcoming the ecological crisis".

In the 1960s and 70s, the use of smoked DMT from crystals—whose production was taught in books and magazines—became popular, at one point ranking among the favorite drugs of psychedelic guru Timothy Leary.

But it was the so-called ayahuasca effect, obtained by combining DMT with inhibitors, that Ott would devote much of his effort to through self-experimentation, guided by the goal of creating analogues of the brew not only to popularize the entheogen but also to reduce pressure on natural populations of Amazonian chacruna and mariri vine, and to mitigate the cultural destruction that ayahuasca tourism could induce in remote communities in Peru, for example.

In this process, Ott settled on Syrian rue as a source of inhibitors, among hundreds of plant species containing these alkaloids, and on black jurema, despite the existence of many other plants that produce them. Syrian rue proved much more efficient than mariri, as its seeds contain 2% to 7% beta-carbolines (inhibitors), compared to 0.45% in the vine. The jurema wine samples analyzed, in turn, contained between 1.25 and 6.5 times more DMT than tested portions of daime. The psychonaut devoted three dozen trials with his own body and mind to scrutinize the doses at which each substance and their combinations produced psychedelic effects, concluding that fifteen grams of ground *Peganum harmala* seeds boiled for an hour with 30% lemon juice were already psychoactive, regardless of association with DMT, though without inducing visions—only mild sedation, buzzing, and a trembling sensation. He found something similar with black jurema, after ruling out the version that passion fruit included in some recipes for the entheogenic wine of the Northeast could be the source of inhibitor: the traditional brew itself would indeed be psychedelic, depending on the amount ingested and not on components kept secret by Indigenous people. His argument: there is a possibility that some unknown MAO inhibitor exists in black jurema. As Ott wrote in the article "Pharmahuasca, Anahuasca, and Vinho da Jurema": "In any case, it is evident there is no lost or missing ingredient, and vinho da jurema is potently visionary by itself, prepared in the traditional manner, and assuming an adequate dose."[12]

In 1997, around the same time he produced juremahuasca for Yatra, Ott stated that the most commonly used source of DMT for the brew spreading through the psychonautic scene was the root bark of black jurema. The following year, it became evident in an interview that his enthusiasm for the alternative entheogen was the origin of an entrepreneurial surge that would engage him in several commercial ventures, such as the founding of the company Pharmacophilia in the Netherlands. For him, it was simply civil disobedience, the sacred democratic duty when a government is rogue, because one can truly see clearly that they have a very malevolent, unethical, anti-ecological, antieconomic, racist, defective, and flawed policy.

In his visionary conception, what he called psychopharmacological engineering would become the world's largest new industry, giving rise to the Microsoft of the psychocosmos. The window of opportunity, he predicted, would remain open for ten years. More than a quarter of a century has passed since this prophecy, which, however, has yet to be fulfilled, although the so-called Psychedelic Renaissance has taken off in the last decade, with consciousness-altering compounds struggling to obtain official regulation for therapeutic use against mental disorders—not exactly the entheogenic revolution envisioned by Ott and so many psychonauts.

On the other hand, the inner divinity that these substances would allow one to glimpse and, perhaps, save the world, from the perspective of someone who lived through the counterculture, does not generate in him a powerful metaphysical conviction. When questioned by Beifuss and Hanna in the 1998 interview about his belief in God, Ott makes explicit the tension between reason and faith, saying that he truly lacks the latter, though he also does not harbor disbelief and declares he does not care about it. In fact, Ott admits never having had visions of entities in a parallel, more fundamental, or truer reality, as some mystics claim. He believes that the universe is our creator, and the divine is the universe itself, with neither science nor religion able to explain its origin. "It's unknowable. I haven't experienced it as plant-spirits, and so I can't vouch for that particular way of seeing it," he says in the interview. "I have to admit that that is possible. And it's certainly plausible. And so I try not to believe in anything, but the other side of that coin is not to disbelieve in anything either."

The Pineal Hypothesis as a Receiver Antenna for Parallel Realities

Jonathan Ott's metaphysical reluctance contrasts with Richard Strassman's embrace of it in *DMT: The Spirit Molecule*, not coincidentally published in Brazil by an ayahuasca church, the Centro Espírita Beneficente União do Vegetal (UDV). Another striking difference between works by the marginal chemist, such as *Pharmacotheon*, and that of physician and university professor Strassman lies in who serves as the subject of phenomenological experimentation with the drug: while Ott recounts what he felt in his own flesh, his more illustrious partner in popularizing DMT among psychonauts bases his speculations on the reports of dozens of volunteers he recruited for his experiments. The researcher himself refuses to disclose whether he has ever been under the influence of the spirit molecule, as Strassman made clear by dodging a direct question from David Jay Brown.[13] This attitude is related to the achievement attained by Strassman, who managed to conduct studies with a psychedelic compound in an academic institution at the height of prohibitionist hegemony, thus needing to maintain or simulate strict detachment from his research subject.

A biology graduate from Stanford University, Strassman recounts in the book that in 1982 he completed a one-year specialization in psychopharmacology at the University of California, San Diego. One day, while walking through the corridors of the city's Veterans Hospital, he mustered the courage to tell his supervisor about his interest in the pineal gland and the role it might play in the secretion of endogenous DMT, that is, produced by the human brain itself, as had been established by Juan Saavedra and Julius Axelrod in 1972.[13] Dr. K., as he appears in the book, immediately stopped walking and turned, serious, stating in a peremptory manner that the pineal had nothing to do with psychedelic drugs.

When asked about the function of DMT in the brain, or why it is produced in the human body, the first hypothesis was that it caused mental illnesses, such as psychosis, which was eventually ruled out. Strassman then set out to find corroboration for his own answer: Because DMT is the spirit molecule. A spirit molecule, he asserts, must reliably elicit certain "spiritual" psychological states. Such states are characterized by feelings of extraordinary happiness, timelessness, and the certainty that what is being experienced is more real than reality. A substance of this kind would be capable of leading one to accept the coexistence of opposites, such as life and death, good and evil; to a knowledge that consciousness continues after death, to a deeper understanding of the primordial unity of all phenomena and a sense of wisdom or love permeating all existence. A spirit molecule would also lead to spiritual realms, or domains that are usually invisible to us and our instruments, inaccessible to our ordinary state of consciousness.

Strassman received his medical training at the Albert Einstein College of Medicine at Yeshiva University in New York, where he was struck by the near-total absence of references to psychedelic substances. He found an opportunity to reopen this field of research at the University of New Mexico, where, at the end of 1988, he submitted a request to the human research ethics committee to study DMT. It took a year and a half to obtain all the necessary federal licenses from the DEA (illicit drugs) and FDA (pharmaceuticals) agencies, allowing him to legally order the substance at the required purity for human experimental use. DMT was ultimately synthesized by David Nichols at Purdue University, with the first five-gram batch delivered in July 1990. Several more months of testing and bureaucracy passed before

Strassman was able to administer the first dose of DMT to a volunteer, on November 19, making him the first researcher in the United States to conduct a clinical trial with a psychedelic substance using public funding since their prohibition during the height of the War on Drugs.

Between 1990 and 1995, Strassman gave approximately four hundred doses of DMT to 55 volunteers on the University of New Mexico campus in Albuquerque. In his book, he recounts his surprise at how frequently participants reported encounters with conscious beings resembling clowns, reptiles, mantises, bees, and spiders. He decided to take these reports seriously, or at least neutrally, rather than trying to convince the participants that the apparitions were merely products of their minds—something they vehemently denied. His approach was akin to that of an anthropologist: Indigenous cultures regularly interact with inhabitants of the invisible landscape and have no difficulty building bridges between these two worlds, he explained.

From this point on, *DMT: The Spirit Molecule* decidedly ventures into metaphysical territory. Strassman compares the normal state of the brain to a TV set tuned to a single channel (objective reality, as it is called, the Normal Channel), whereas the effect of DMT would be akin to switching stations and tuning into other planes of existence. From this metaphor, he moves into pure speculation, as he himself admits, but many—among psychonauts and esotericists—take his science-tinged fantasy literally. "I claim little understanding of the physics underlying theories of parallel universes and dark matter. What I do know, however, causes me to consider them as possible places where DMT might lead us, once we have rushed past the personal," he speculates. "DMT may allow our receiver brain to sense these multiverses."

"DMT is the cosmos in a little cup," Rodrigo Grünewald might say of Rick Strassman's metaphysical speculations. The Brazilian researcher, however, criticizes the sacralization of the molecule promoted by the American scientist and naively embraced by urban neo-shamanism—people more interested in the chemical effect than in tradition and coherence. He also takes issue with the unreflective trivialization of the notion of the sacred, as in the contemporary rebranding of Catimbó as Jurema Sagrada: "I don't like the name. Have you ever seen Sacred Hinduism? Sacred Catholicism?" He notes, however, that he understands the political motivation, centered in Recife and Olinda, to destigmatize this form of religiosity that has been rendered invisible, providing a less prejudiced designation both within and outside the Northeast of Brazil. Today, on the other hand, he views positively the constant movement of Jurema Sagrada between the semi-arid backlands and the rainforest zone along the coast, where the plant and the drink acquired their

Indigenous Tupi name (something like "yu-rema," full of thorns), allowing the entity Malunguinho to be celebrated both at festivals with hundreds or thousands of people in the forest zone of Abreu e Lima and in Atikum ceremonies in Indigenous huts in the backlands of Carnaubeira da Penha. For the anthropologist, the ritual is as important as, or even more important than, the entheogen itself.

His former student Estêvão Palitot agrees. Guided by Grünewald, he attended rituals held in the mud huts of the Atikum, with jurema wine prepared without Syrian rue or any other obvious source of inhibitors, in which an alternate reality is glimpsed—one as real as the real world, at least from the anthropological perspective. "They create a world. Each of these groups is a creator of cultural realities," he says. "This spirituality is present all the time. The entheogen may simply be the broad, unobstructed channel."

Born into a very religious family, both Catholic and Kardecist, Palitot has taken ayahuasca, jurema wine, and juremahuasca. Like his mentor Grünewald, he has seen souls (spirits) pass before him, all of them overcome by pain and disorientation, but he fears them neither emotionally nor scientifically. He has witnessed "pretos velhos" (African ancestors) and anthropomorphic entities, experienced spirit possession, and, in a UDV session, felt a vine stem sprouting from his insides and coming out of his mouth, leaving an earthy aftertaste. But neither for this reason he believes he is missing something as an intellectual; on the contrary, as he made clear in several parts of the conversation. To do science, one must be open to this imaginary dimension, he reflects: "If you are not, you see some things; if you are, you see those things and a few others as well." "Who am I to say that mermaids do not exist?" asks Grünewald, his mentor and friend. "Those who only think about molecules believe that the others [juremeiros] are making up fairy tales."

Notes

1. Most of the biographical information on Rodrigo de Azeredo Grünewald was obtained through interviews conducted in Rio de Janeiro on April 28, 2022, and in Campina Grande on March 21, 2023. Other information comes from his book *Jurema* (Mercado de Letras, 2020).
2. Rodrigo de Azeredo Grünewald, *"Regime de índio" e faccionalismo: os Atikum da Serra do Umã.* PPGAS/MN/UFRJ, 1993. Master's thesis.
3. Interview on March 21, 2023.

4. "Contribuições das Tradições da Jurema para o Campo da Saúde Mental." Available at: < https://www.youtube.com/live/OaiIrKIa6wM?si=154F-5z_YH4SnNXR > . Accessed: December 20, 2024.

5. Jonathan Ott, *Hallucinogenic Plants of North America.* Berkeley: Wingbow Press, 1976.

6. Jonathan Ott, *Pharmacotheon: Drogas enteógenas, sus fuentes vegetales y su historia.* Barcelona: La Liebre de Marzo, 1996.

7. "Contribuições das Tradições da Jurema para o Campo da Saúde Mental." Available at: < https://www.youtube.com/live/OaiIrKIa6wM?si=154F-5z_YH4SnNXR > . Accessed: December 20, 2024.

8. Rodrigo Grünewald, *Jurema.* Campinas: Mercado de Letras, 2020. p. 132.

9. Marcos Alexandre dos Santos Albuquerque, *Destreza e Sensibilidade: Os Vários Sujeitos da Jurema (As Práticas Rituais e os Diversos Usos de um Enteógeno Nordestino)* Campina Grande/ PB: UFCG, 2002. Undergraduate thesis. p. 85.

10. Will Beifuss and Jon Hanna, "Jonathan Ott Speaks..." Part 1. *The Entheogen Review*, v. 8, n. 1., pp. 25–34, 1999.

11. David Jay Brown, "An Interview with Rick Strassman," in Frontiers of Psychedelic Consciousness: Conversations with Albert Hofmann, Stanislav Grof, Rick Strassman, Jeremy Narby, Simon Posford, and Others. Rochester, VT /Toronto: Park Street Press, 2015. p. 151.

12. Jonathan Ott. "Pharmahuasca, Anahuasca and Vinho da Jurema: Human Pharmacology of Oral DMT plus Harmine". In: Christian Rätsch, John R. Baker, Claudia Müller-Ebeling (Eds.). Jahrbuch für Ethnomedizin und Bewusstseinsforschung / Yearbook for Ethnomedicine and Consciousness 1997/98. Berlim: Verlag für Wissenschaft und Bildung, 2000.

13. Juan Saavedra and Julius Axelrod, "A specific and sensitive enzymatic assay for tryptamine in tissues." *Journal of Pharmacology and Experimental Therapeutics*, v. 182, n. 3, pp. 363–9, September 1, 1972.

Changa and DMT Crystals, Engines of Cosmopolitan Neo-Shamanism

My first direct contact with DMT from black jurema did not occur through juremahuasca, but rather in the form of vaporized crystals heated in a glass pipe. This inaugural experience took place at a neo-shamanic festival, Equinox, held during the week of the autumn equinox, in the last days of March in the Southern Hemisphere, on Algodões beach, in southern Bahia.

Before the ceremony in which I inhaled DMT, Claudia and I had participated in a beautiful ritual under the full moon of March 18, 2022, two days before the planetary event when day and night are of exactly equal length.[1] The fire ceremony begins at sunset at Matinha, a house nestled in the Atlantic Rainforest, around a bonfire with logs arranged according to the cardinal points, an altar with fruit, candles, and an image of Our Lady. About twenty participants take part in the ritual, which lasts eight hours, receiving from a Mexican healer a stick and a strand of red wool, or more than on strand if necessary. They tie a knot for each person with whom they have had sexual relations, mentally offer thanks, wrap the wool around the stick, and, one by one, circle the fire counterclockwise to throw the object into the flames.

After many prayers, songs, speeches, and tears, a young man kneels before the fire and asks permission to share something personal. He clenches his hands below his navel and speaks of the tightness that afflicts him. His expression intensifies: tremors, crying, sweating, contortions, sighs, screams, howls. Prostrate, he buries his face in the sand and stretches his arms toward the fire. The tension in the circle of celebrants rises; the young man seems drawn to the flames. To the right, another young man stands and takes charge of what appears to be a possession: he embraces the distressed youth, runs his hand over him and sprinkles water on his head, blows and kisses his tormented

M. Leite, *The Psychedelic Science of the Jurema Tree*, Copernicus Books, https://doi.org/10.1007/978-3-032-22705-8_6

face, whispers words in his ear. Someone starts a song to Oxum, the orixá of fresh water. Several women, who make the majority of attendants around the fire, stand and join the embrace. Everyone sings together, while the young man calms down to the repeated words "love" and "joy," eventually smiling and giving thanks.

The ceremony continues until 2:30 a.m. Other rituals will begin from 5 a.m.—meditation, yoga, sacred feminine and masculine, constellations, and detox. There are experiences with power plants and substances, such as ayahuasca, tobacco, and cacao. The Equinox Festival, which had opened five days earlier, brought together about forty people on the Bahia beach of the Maraú peninsula and would officially end only the following Sunday.

Neo-shamanism, or urban shamanism, runs like an underground river beneath the solid ground of established religions. Its hallmark is eclecticism, more than syncretism, for the mystical kaleidoscope does not form a recognizable doctrine that coordinates elements from other faiths. It is plural, fluid, flexible, open to any form of spirituality, unconcerned with consistency. At the festivals, there is room for Mexican *Abuelos*, crystals, orixás, Umbanda caboclos, tarot cards, Tibetan mantras, odes to Jurema, and Santo Daime hymns. Participants are members of a cosmopolitan tribe, the children and grandchildren of the New Age, who identify themselves by the individual pursuit of wellness and its synonyms—healing, harmony, balance, happiness, love, compassion, divine light, transcendence, peace. It does not matter where they come from or what they believe in, but that they are willing to chant in unison: "May all beings be blessed, may they feel the purest love in their hearts, may all be enlightened by the light of truth and live in peace, harmony, and prosperity." Or else sing under the tipi of Casa del Mar, a cone of logs four- or five-meters high evoking the ceremonial tents of American indigenous peoples:

> *Jurema, oh juremá*
> *Jurema, oh juremá*
> *I was in the forest with my arrow in hand*
> *And Mother Jurema inside my heart*
> *And there in the forest I met Tupinambá*
> *And Mother Jurema to accompany me*
> *Jurema, oh juremá*
> *Jurema, oh juremá*
> *It was there in the forest that I found inspiration*
> *To follow the path of the heart.*

All translations of lyrics, verses and quotes from Portuguese to English are the author's with help of AI

Anyone can become a pajé or guru. What is revered there is the abstract figure of the shaman, not the healer or sorcerer of specific peoples and cultures from Siberia or Latin America, the sacred woman or man of flesh and blood who performs blessings or divination according to strict rituals. These are fleeting collectives, coagulated for a single encounter, not a community formed by ties of blood, unique myths, and cosmology. They have little in common with traditional shamanism as studied by Mircea Eliade, for example. Many among Brazilian neo-shamanists share a common origin in the ayahuasca-based religions, such as Santo Daime, Barquinha, and União do Vegetal. This tradition, which emerged in twentieth-century Amazonia, is itself marked by syncretism, as it reconciles elements of Amerindian rites and beliefs (beginning with the psychedelic brew), Christian, African, and Kardecist influences. It is a mysticism that is theologically porous and adaptable to different cultures, localities, and religious conceptions, allowing for varied forms of arrangement and bricolage of beliefs. In times of existential disarray, with politics degraded into childish antics on social media, precarious work relations, fragmented identities, a planet's climate in turmoil, threatening pandemics, renewed war, and temples sold off, a spirituality of great resonance emerges for urban middle-class professionals, squeezed to the bone by the corporate machine.

At Equinox, several women had the same story to tell: disillusioned with their careers—even if successful and often incompatible with motherhood—they gave up everything and chose a simple life on the coast of Bahia for themselves and their children. This was the case for Alessandra Rossi, who left a good job at a software company to run the guesthouse Na Villa dos Algodões and become one of the festival's organizers, alongside the Spaniard Amaya Arguedas, from Casa del Mar, and Gabi Pimienta. It was also the case for Michelle "Tukiama" Button, a Mexican who led the fire ceremony and had interrupted her career in public relations for luxury brands to begin practicing with the Wixarika people and their peyote cactus (*Lophophora williamsii*), which they call *hikuri*.

In Brazil, dozens of Indigenous peoples use ayahuasca ceremonially. Just as the ayahuasca religions learned from them the method of preparing the tea, mixing in the cauldron the ingredients of extra-forest cults and doctrines, the neo-shamanics have distanced themselves from these churches, retaining only a few of their anchors, such as the simple and beautiful hymns of the Santo Daime tradition, while incorporating fragments of religious and mystical practices from all over, from North America to Africa and Asia. The prototypical figure of the shaman, however, is no longer that of the northern Asian sorcerer who gave rise to the now-globalized term—people with the power to heal, visit the dead, fly to other dimensions, and foresee the future in trance, a role originally studied among the Siberian Chukchi and Koryak peoples. Now, a generic Amerindian pajé prevails, a kind of collective reminiscence of initiation into the power of ayahuasca that so many of these seekers of balance went to find in the forests of Acre and Amazonas states in Brazil, or Peru. There is also room for healers from Central and North America who use "magic" mushrooms with psilocybin and the peyote cactus with mescaline to travel between worlds.

One may debate whether this eclecticism, by neglecting what is specific and sacred in each people's rituals, amounts to cultural appropriation. Yet this would be equivalent to anthropological purism, failing to recognize that these peoples have already engaged in the globalized ayahuasca circuit, traveling to Brazilian capitals and other countries to present their shamanic practices, cosmologies, and medicines to those able to pay for these "experiences"—even if payment is often euphemistically referred to as an "exchange of energy."

In a lecture at the Equinox Festival, Paulo de Azevedo, or Purna Chandra, presented the Vibra Quantum treatment system, invoking "metacognition"— in his concept, the need for each person to become aware of what they do not know about themselves in order to heal and break the patterns of behavior, explanation, and reaction in which so many find themselves trapped. Nothing new for those who have undergone psychotherapy, but also nothing new for neuroscientists and psychiatrists who understand depression, for example, as an overactive default mode network in the brain, culminating in the rumination of negative thoughts that can lead to prostration and suicidal ideation. For some, at least, a molecule such as DMT may open the way to new neural connections and other ways of facing problems, provided the drug is consumed in a supportive context.

This was Purna's proposal for the final day's experience at Equinox. Dressed in white, with a dot painted on his forehead, he set up in the Oca—a large oval shelter in the forest at Casa del Mar—an altar with crystals, bottles of scented water, tarot cards, stones, feathers, incense, and oriental bells. Prominently displayed were three bottles of ayahuasca from different sources, for the first three phases of the work, four in total. After the first dose, or "dispatch," each participant was to focus on self-knowledge, reflecting on what, in the previous year, had sparked their curiosity, sadness, anger, fear, joy, and enthusiasm. In the second phase, the focus was on insights, current challenges, and recently closed or opened cycles. In the third, the celebration phase, one should establish short- and long-term goals, creating images to anchor these objectives. The fourth phase is dedicated to relaxation and download, without the distribution of the beverage, in which a maracá (ceremonial rattle) is passed from hand to hand, giving each person the opportunity to speak about what they experienced during the previous six hours of concentration.

The first ayahuasca, brownish-yellow in color and fermented, made a hissing sound as gas escaped from the bottle when opened. The loudspeakers began to play an eclectic playlist—indigenous melodies, Hindu tunes, and also Santo Daime hymns, such as "Divine Light":

> *Divine light, where is my forgiveness*
> *I want to be a child of the Virgin Mother*
> *She is the key to reach Jesus Christ*
> *Divine light, illuminate the darkness*
> *The darkness that dwells within me*
> *And the enemies I keep inside myself*
> *Divine light surrounding your children*
> *Illuminating the path to salvation*
> *Love is the key that opens the first door*
> *And the second opens with forgiveness*
> *To pass through, this door is very narrow*
> *But once inside, it is a great hall*
> *Divine light, only love and forgiveness*
> *Only truly, only if it comes from the heart*
> *Divine light, I want to see your radiance*
> *For this child is already weary of the darkness*

Still responding to the first questionnaire that Purna had proposed to sharpen concentration, I began to feel the force of the daime arriving. I meditated alternately sitting and lying down. I was repeatedly moved, with tears of joy welling up as I sang the innocent lyrics of the simple hymns, with the familiar sobs that rise in the throat when music uplifts, and as I heard Purna moving through the hall, singing with his free, nasal voice, shaking feathers, sprinkling scented water and incense smoke over the psychonauts present. I noticed that I could better control my feelings and tears when I articulated the lyrics and sang out loud, letting the emotion out instead of swallowing it for fear of others' judgment.

At the second serving of ayahuasca, Purna asked me not to get up to be served the tea when the bell rang. We had agreed to fulfill my wish to experience the power of black jurema, replacing the drink distributed to everyone with a pipe full of DMT crystals extracted from the root of the *Mimosa tenuiflora* tree. At his request, Daniel, who has extensive experience with DMT and changa, came over to my mat, kneeling beside me. He was shirtless, revealing his tattooed torso, and looked at me with his clear, intense eyes, holding in his hand the glass pipe he called the "device." Under the effect of anticipation, my heart was pounding, racing. He asked if I had ever smoked DMT (no) and if I could inhale the smoke without coughing and hold it for six seconds (maybe). I could take up to three puffs in a row, but I was not to worry: The medicine is self-dosing, he said, and I would know when to stop and would feel the need to lie down.

So it was. On the second puff, I signaled that I would stop and stretched out on the mat. My vision filled with volutes and arabesques in predominantly pink tones, as if entering a fantastic mosque. I tasted an ultra-vegetal flavor in my mouth, unlike anything I had ever experienced. The tip of my tongue and the part of my lips where the pipe had touched became numb, as if under the effect of jambu, the anesthetic herb used in Amazonian cuisine. An extremely powerful, uplifting impact. I lay there for a long time, or so it seemed, my chest full of strong and positive feelings—love, compassion, communion, fellowship, empathy—not all the synonyms in the world could adequately describe what was overflowing. The breeze on my body was friendly, a caressing source of pleasure. The incense and scented waters were delicious to the nose, almost colorful in their intensity. I felt a deep identification with the hymns, but, curiously, few articulated thoughts connected to the emotions, which I only managed to write down four days later, already back in São Paulo, still under the afterglow of that dazzling light.

When the bell sounded for the third phase of the Vibra Quantum session, Purna did not serve me the same ayahuasca as the others, but rather the one in a colorful bottle, a very dark, almost black liquid that left sediment at the bottom of the cup and a terrible bitter aftertaste in my mouth. The prevailing silence of phases one and two gave way to a bit of everything in phases three (celebration) and four (integration). A mother danced with her small children, couples embraced, friends cried together, strangers kissed, tears flowed with the songs or under the scented water that Purna sprinkled from time to time over those meditating sitting or lying down, at the height of the ayahuasca's effect. A stubborn atheist, I found myself immersed in gratitude for the simple gifts of that circle and of nature. People danced and sang, celebrating the fact of coming together and suspending judgment about everything, accepting without fear whatever appeared before their eyes, open or closed. I entered the ceremony with determination, danced, embraced with Claudia and the Mexican healer Tukiama, and told her she was "mi hermanita desde siempre," which made her laugh. "We have finally met," I added. I hugged Daniel and thanked him for introducing me to DMT from black jurema.

The only vision I had during the seven hours of work was the round face of my unborn granddaughter, Marina, to whom I promised more calm and patience than I had shown her brother, Antônio, and cousins Alice and Tomás. In Purna's third questionnaire, I wrote down that after finishing this book, I would face the long-postponed challenge of writing fiction. And, perhaps, study singing. In the fourth part of the ceremony, the only one not preceded by a dose of ayahuasca, I was the third to receive the maracá and the word. I thanked Alessandra and Amaya for their hospitality, and Tukiama and Purna for the transporting sessions. I said it had been an afternoon of many tears, most of them shed for joy and communion. I hugged Tukiama and Paulo tightly in farewell. The Frenchwoman Sara came to us, the oldest couple there, saying she saw much of her own parents in us, and we kissed. "*Merci beaucoup*," I recalled from the memory of the boy who had attended the early years of elementary school at Lycée Pasteur in São Paulo. Claudia and I walked back to the inn along the beach, hand in hand and happy, under the full moon.

Autonomy of Healing with Juremas from Brazil and Acacias from Australia

The psychoanalyst Paulo de Azevedo received the name Purna Chandra by the grace of guru Purushatraya Swami, during his first initiation in Bhakti Yoga. Today, he uses ayahuasca more frequently in his work, but he has extensive experience with changa and pure DMT crystals extracted from black jurema. He was 47 years old when I visited him at his property near Pium beach, in Parnamirim (state of Rio Grande do Norte) a neighboring municipality of Natal, in March 2023, six months after the Vibra Quantum ceremony in Algodões. As soon as he finished his jiu-jitsu training with instructor Antônio Almeida on the spacious terrace of his house, he showed me the large pot in which he prepares ayahuasca in a clearing near the adjacent creek, where the tree canopies close in, forming what he calls a natural oca (as Indigenous peoples in Brazil call their collective houses), the place where he also conducts his group sessions. He does not like to be called a neo-shaman, as his professional goal is to bring well-being to his clients, not necessarily to awaken their spirituality. To develop his Vibra Quantum system, he says he dedicated himself to studying quantum mechanics and psychoanalysis, but today he goes beyond the issues of transference between analyst and analysand and healing through words, resorting to musical vibrations and the powerful tool of ayahuasca.

It was music, in fact, that led him to psychedelia. Raised in Belo Horizonte, he accompanied his father from a young age on record-buying trips to the Hi-Fi store at a shopping mall. At eleven, he entered the store alone and left with records by Led Zeppelin and AC/DC, becoming a devoted fan of psychedelic rock. At fourteen, he got his first mixer to create and listen to music in his room, but soon began performing as a DJ at family parties and, later, professionally. He even played at festivals such as Skol Beats and Universo Paralello. In that scene, he has encountered MDMA and LSD, but had difficulty obtaining consciousness modifiers in Belo Horizonte of the 1990s, until he discovered that there was an abundant psychedelic right there, in Santo Daime, and in 2000 he donned the farda (uniform), that is, became a full member of the church.

Around the same time, he was introduced to black jurema at a rave by his friend Daniel Strickland (the same Daniel who had initiated me in Algodões). Daniel gave him a small vial of crystals and a glass pipe, along with instructions on how to dose and use it. He started with half a dose, found the effect similar to ayahuasca, and jumped to one and a half doses. "The altar in my room turned into an amusement park, a roller coaster taking over the entire space," he described. "The car stopped and picked me up, showing me things I didn't even know existed. I need to get to know this substance better," he concluded at the time. "It's like putting on a new pair of glasses," he said in the interview under the trees of his natural oca in Pium, covered by the flowers of his patterned black shirt and the tattoo on his right arm, comparing DMT visions to the discovery of a new way of seeing life.

The use of DMT at electronic music or neo-shamanic festivals, not exactly spiritual, faces restrictions from traditional shamanism of Indigenous origin and from established ayahuasca religions. It is often pejoratively labeled as "recreational" use, or condemned as "entheotainment," a neologism coined to stigmatize those who mix supposedly sacred entheogens with entertainment. The prejudice is directed especially against DMT crystals and changa, which are dismissed as "smokable ayahuasca" or "ayahuasca crack."[2] This form of consumption can trigger an immediate psychedelic experience (taking effect within seconds) that is brief (generally 10 to 15 min), thus dispensing with the six-hour or longer rituals and the purges (vomiting, diarrhea) and strict diets that often precede them.

The chemist Jonathan Ott rejects this view as shamanic neo-calvinism and, while honoring South American and Asian shamans as kindred spirits to contemporary scientists in their pharmacognostic experimentation, advocates for the democratization of this accumulated knowledge by justifying his efforts to create analogues of ayahuasca such as juremahuasca. In an article, he wrote that he wished to help people circumvent the prohibition of entheogens and the attempts by modern Santo Daime religious groups to co-opt and monopolize shamanic technology, which he sees as a common heritage of all humanity. He thus set out to enable people to prepare a potent entheogen in the comfort and safety of their own homes, using legal and harmless herbs that grow on every continent and in most ecosystems.[3] Ott takes pride in having disseminated a recipe worldwide that introduced black jurema to the international psychedelic market in 1996, and at one point made it the main source of DMT for psychonauts. In his view, only misanthropes and die-hard Calvinists could oppose the pursuit of pleasure with the help of entheogens: "Pleasure, enjoyment, is the best medicine against whatsoever malaise of the spirit, and it is always good for any ills or infirmities of the body."[4]

Like Ott, Graham St John of Griffith University in Australia, in addition to neo-shamanic and gnostic applications (self-knowledge and enlightenment), defends in the article "Aussiewaska"[5] the recreational use of changa, which he claims is an Australian invention. It is said to have arisen from the efforts of a vibrant psychonaut community seeking not the healing promised by ayahuasca churches, but what might be called grace, in a non-religious sense: a liminal state capable of shattering social conditioning and amplifying visionary experiences, catapulting travelers into a fearful and wondrous hyperspace, both affirmative and subversive, private and accelerated, in contrast to the ceremonial and purgative trance of traditional ayahuasca. For St John, losing control of the mind is essential for healing, but it seems paradoxical that at the same time control is surrendered to others, to authority figures in churches or shamanic circles, in clear contradiction to the libertarian and anarchist impulse of the counterculture.

Instead of black jurema, the preferred source of DMT in Australia is the 150 species of acacias found in the country. In the original changa recipe created by Julian Palmer in 2003, the dimethyltryptamine extracted primarily from the branches and leaves of *Acacia obtusifolia* is combined with inhibitors from the mariri vine native to the Amazon. The mixture results in a smokable product that serves to moderate the radical experience produced when vaporizing pure DMT crystals, which can overwhelm the psychonaut and induce aversion to repeating the journey. The blend with mariri is also said to extend the effect to somewhere between twenty and thirty minutes. As changa spread through the Australian psychedelic scene, it acquired new versions, with the addition of herbs and leaves such as passionfruit, mint, blue lotus, lemon, lavender, peppermint, Syrian rue, and pau d'arco. From Australia, "smokable ayahuasca" would spread around the world. According to St John, however, in Brazil changa rarely contains shavings of ayahuasca mariri, and in fact the

DMT I tried at the Equinox festival did not include an inhibitor, nor even herbs, just crystals obtained from black jurema.

To illustrate what he called "psychedelic theophany," which he sees as distant from the religious life of ayahuasca churches and equally from what is disparaged within them as entheotainment, St John cites the tryptamine visions of an attendee at the 2009 Glade festival in the United Kingdom, who even considered founding a Psytrance religion:

> [...] the most amazing alien beings dancing, flirting at me, a couple kissing and exploding into a flood of multicolored tessellated tiled fragments, the Egyptian sun god Horus erupting from a foam of seething fractals. I saw Homer Simpson eating a doughnut and cathedrals of extreme beauty and color. It was the most amazing 15 minutes of my life! Far better than any CGI visuals or computer graphics could generate..[6]

St John notes that such "Disneyfication" of the entheogenic hyperspace intensifies the discontent of those who lament the commercialization of changa as the ayahuasca -crack, but the author doubts that it could ever be properly categorized as a recreational drug, given its capacity to shatter illusions and reveal the core of things—an experience that may not be enjoyable. "Purist [ayahuasca] drinkers are typically suspicious of DMT users—who lack a certain legitimacy, if not virtue, so far removed from the cultural and theologically sanctioned traditions of brews and snuffs." Critics especially resent the notion that changa represents a more evolved stage of ayahuasca and the implicit suggestion that the DMT from chacruna is the most important component of the brew, to the detriment of the no less sacred substances provided by the vine. What Ott and St John celebrate as the universal sharing of shamanic technology, traditionalists see as the cultural appropriation of ancestral knowledge for inappropriate purposes.

Anthropologist Esther Jean Langdon, from the Federal University of Santa Catarina in Brazil, points out that Amazonian shamanism, with its central metaphors of predation and cannibalism, is far from gentle. She disagrees with the notion that shamanism is a faithful translation of pure Amerindian cultures for non-Indigenous people,[7] preferring instead the idea of dialogue and collective construction in response to the tragedy that the arrival of Europeans represented for countless peoples whose diverse practices, in fact, are difficult to fit into an ideal type created by anthropology to describe religiosity studied on other continents. Not even the idea of a mestizo shamanism, such as that which emerged from interactions between forest groups and colonial cities that consumed pajelanças (Indigenous rituals), would suffice to subsume urban religions like Santo Daime, which, nevertheless, claim to be heirs of authentic, original Indigenous traditions, even as they participate in globalized networks of entheogen and belief exchange. It would be more appropriate to speak of shamanisms, plural, which in any case would provide no grounds to disqualify neo-shamans or white shamans as lacking authentic credentials and roots.

"Native shamanisms today must be regarded as the product of the colonial encounter, as many authors have argued [...] and not an archaic religion from the past," she argues. "Specific focus on witchcraft has indicated that the dark, non-loving aspects of shamanism are important strategies in this encounter [...] in which urban and mestizo shamanisms express the concerns of the subaltern classes in a capitalist economy." In place of the shamans' flights between worlds, possession is increasingly important as the essence of trance, as is the incorporation of African elements, rhythms, and animism into rituals, alongside Catholic saints. The urban poor prioritize in their demand's afflictions related to love, illness, bad luck, unemployment, business, and other sources of misfortune. From this perspective, festival-goers, generally middle-class people, are not so different from the poor who once flocked to Catimbó ceremonies in Alhandra or to ayahuasca sessions in the Amazon and today mingle with wealthier people in Jurema Sagrada terreiros or Santo Daime churches: all are seeking transcendence and relief with the help of entheogens, whether ayahuasca, jurema wine, changa, or pure DMT crystals. And it will not be by claiming doctrines or traditions considered more true or authentic that one will succeed in disqualifying as degeneration or cultural appropriation the reinvention of shamanic technologies that different Amerindian peoples have been exchanging among themselves for millennia in their struggle to remain alive, healthy, and, indeed, Indigenous.

The Mobilization of Entheogens Against Colonial Thought in the University

For the Indigenous peoples of Northeastern Brazil, at the epicenter of this effort at self-preservation is a power plant, black jurema. However, it is a mistake to imagine that the resistance associated with the entheogens of jurema wine is a thing of the distant colonial past, buried in the poorly documented memory of santidades and Indigenous or quilombola revolts. Nor would it be correct to conclude that jurema fulfilled its role in the reemergence, in the 1980s, of Northeastern ethnic groups who proved their own "Indianness" to the Indigenous affairs agency FUNAI by dancing torés and drinking the wine, and that after this the cult surrounding this tree lost its importance. The fact that this religiosity remains almost ignored by academic institutions and by the population of other regions of Brazil, when not outright scorned, does not invalidate the prominent role it still plays in articulating demands for land regularization (demarcation and recognition of Indigenous lands), health promotion, and cultural survival, as I was able to witness at the 7th Gathering of Shamans, Midwives, and Holders of Traditional Indigenous Knowledge of Pernambuco, in October 2023, in the Kambiwá territory of the municipality of Ibimirim.

At the meeting held in the Baixa da Alexandra village, there are representatives from almost all twelve ethnic groups present in the backlands of Pernambuco, who have the use of black jurema as one of the most distinctive common elements among them. After several rounds of the toré in the sandy courtyard, everyone enters the oca to the intense sound of maracás and the sweet smoke of campiôs, the conical pipes characteristic of these peoples. A young Xucuru, adopting the gestures of someone embodying an African ancestor (slurred, rustic speech, hunched torso, bulging eyes), takes the microphone and leads the chorus: "Hail the Sacred Jurema! Hail the pretos velhos! Hail spirituality!" Everyone then sings the chant "Hail the Sacred Jurema":

> *I am a **child** of Jurema*
> *I come from the land of Jurema*
> *I will call my caboclos*
> *To come and work*

Shortly after lunch, I find a group of Pankará beside the oca drinking the dark beverage kept in a plastic Fanta bottle, served in a gourd, and they confirm it is wine made from black jurema. They offer me the drink; I ask if I am allowed to partake, not being Indigenous (naively thinking that my slightly dark skin might lead them to mistake me for one of them), and the oldest man, holding the bottle, fills the gourd to the brim and extends it toward me. I drink it all in three or four gulps, not removing the gourd from my lips, even though I am bothered by the bitterness and the intense smoky flavor. One of them refuses the wine, claiming he has just eaten, to which I react, a bit alarmed: "So have I!" No noticeable effect appears in the following hours, although even before drinking I was already filled with a sense of peace and contentment at seeing so many people gathered, celebrating and resisting.

The speeches continue over two days, some more bureaucratic, others more visionary and activist. One of the most impassioned is the Pankará Manuel Pedro dos Santos, juremeiro Manezinho, who puts the issue of Indigenous land at the center of the gathering, singing: "I want it demarcated, I want it cleared of invaders,[8] I want it ratified! I have the maracá in hand to wake up Funai and get to work." He is the brother of chief Maria das Dores dos Santos, Dorinha, the first Pankará woman to assume a leadership position and the third in the state of Pernambuco. At 59 years old at the time of the interview, the nursing technician and traditional midwife had already served as a city councilor in Carnaubeira da Penha, led a blockade of the road leading to the city to demand quality Indigenous education, and, in 2024, held the position of Secretary of Indigenous Affairs and Racial Equality in her city. She attributes her strength to having been baptized in Jurema and to the mediumistic abilities that the sacred plant and her cabocla awakened in her as a child. "I was born with the gift, I used to accompany my father and grandfather when they performed the ritual," she says. In 2003, during a Jurema ceremony, she says she received, in a direct message from enchanted beings—something that had previously only happened in dreams—the mission to lead the 5,225 Pankará she reports living on the 15,000 hectares of territory identified in the Arapuá mountains, still awaiting demarcation and ratification in 2024. "They are all my children," says the midwife, who estimates she has helped about 15,000 children to be born.

It is not easy to recognize and untangle the winding thread woven with the roots of black jurema that connects Dorinha to Julian Palmer in Australia, to Rodrigo Grünewald in Campina Grande and Rio, or to Jonathan Ott in the United States and Mexico. Especially because, for this Indigenous people and their relatives in Pernambuco, the psychedelic effect of DMT is the least prominent component of the plant *Mimosa tenuiflora*. The thread will become a little clearer to the reader, I hope, if you know that I became a guest of the Kambiwá in Baixa da Alexandra thanks to the psychologist Alexandre Franca Barreto, a professor at the Federal University of the São Francisco Valley (UNIVASF) in Petrolina (Pernambuco), who, if he does not fit the profile of a neo-shaman, at least qualifies as a psychonaut enthusiastic about jurema.

We met in August 2023 in Vitória (in the southeastern state of Espírito Santo), at the 26th Conference of the International Institute for Bioenergetic Analysis (IIBA), to which I had been invited by therapists Léia Cardenuto and Liane Zink to speak about my book *Psiconautas*. During the coffee break, Barreto enthusiastically—a usual trait in everything he does—shared his experiences with jurema and with Indigenous peoples of the northeastern backlands, precisely the topics I was seeking to explore further for another book. After a few weeks of exchanging messages, he prepared an itinerary for October that would take me not only to Baixa da Alexandra, for the gathering of midwives and shamans, but also to Brejo do Burgo, for the

Festa do Amaro among the Pankararé—and also to a neo-shamanic ceremony with juremahuasca in Petrolina, which stands among the most remarkable psychedelic experiences I have ever had.

Barreto qualifies as a seasoned traveler in many respects, having undertaken an extensive journey through the various worlds that make up Brazil. Born in Recife, his life underwent two major upheavals around the age of two. In the first, he was literally thrown against a glass door by the hammock in which he was swinging with his mother, an accident that left prominent scars on his back and soul. In the second, the family moved to São Paulo so that his father could manage his family's clothing store branch. An artisan and artist who faced racism from his wife's family for being Black, his father accumulated frustrations in business and began to suffer health problems caused by alcohol consumption, such as vertigo that no medication could control. Improvement came only through spiritual means, his son recounts, when he began attending an Umbanda house, Estrela da Paz, and entrusted himself to the care of the "pretos velhos", old Black spirits. Meanwhile, his mother, a geologist trained at the Federal University of Pernambuco, pursued an academic career with a master's and doctorate at the University of São Paulo, studying the paleoenvironment of the Bahia backlands.

The family's return to Recife occurred when Barreto was already an adolescent, during a period of great cultural effervescence, with the mangue beat musical movement at the forefront. He developed a keen interest in psychoactives, was active in a graffiti group, and was "quite a handful." A skeptic, he joined the student movement. The pain persisted; he was unable to form attachments to any woman, sought help in psychotherapy, and spent three months crying through each forty-minute session. Guided by his father, he sought out a temple of the eclectic sect Vale do Amanhecer, which he attended every weekend, and there developed his path of mediumistic study, receiving care from Pai Joaquim de Aruanda, an old Black spirit of Umbanda. It was only at age 23, during his first experience with ayahuasca, that the trauma he had suffered at age two became clear: "I saw everything again as an observer. The scene [of the collision with the glass door] turned into a leaf, then a branch, and a tree with many other memories of my mother, then a forest."

He completed a master's in anthropology, his first of three children was born, and he moved to Petrolina in 2009 after passing a civil service exam for UNIVASF. He grew close to professors working with Indigenous peoples, which piqued his curiosity about the world of Jurema. In 2014, after a seminar on health, education, and spirituality, he came into contact with DMT from black jurema in the form of juremahuasca, a beverage prepared with Syrian rue, during a neo-shamanic ceremony, where he saw many things: "Intoxicating ecstasy, a profound pleasure. I saw the procession in which Jurema was brought, on another planet. The beings merged, with both human and plant characteristics. Vivid and beautiful color. I had a soul encounter with Juracy [Marques]."

At 42 years old at the time of the interview in Petrolina, Barreto holds a doctorate in education, is trained as a bioenergetic analyst, and has made several forays among Indigenous peoples such as the Truká, Pankará, Fulni-ô, and Kapinawá. "I needed the colonial [academic] training to be able to appreciate the richness of ancestral knowledge, of the peoples of the territory and of Africans, and to understand these worldviews." In the decade following his first experience with juremahuasca, he cultivated a friendship with Juracy Marques. Together with him and other daimista friends from Petrolina, he started a neo-shamanic group that regularly drinks the entheogenic beverage at a small farm in the Serra dos Morgados, in Jaguarari (state of Bahia), Marques's hometown, now a professor at the State University of Bahia (UNEB). Thus was born Aldeia Luz da Jurema, which they nicknamed Alma ("soul" in Portuguese).

In the Bahian backlands, Juracy Marques grew up attending a Candomblé terreiro where his mother was a priestess and there was a strong influence of Indigenous spirituality. As a teenager, he studied at a Catholic school and fell in love with the liturgy, became an altar boy determined to become a priest, and learned that Candomblé and Umbanda were supposedly demonic beliefs. He tried to convince his mother, a daughter of Iemanjá, to leave the terreiro life, something that at the time of the interview, at age 46, he would describe as an intrusion, saying that the study of anthropology and psychoanalysis had been a way to distance himself from the Catholic Church, adopt a materialist worldview, and make amends with his mother.

He reconnected with his own Black and Indigenous heritage, as well as with Candomblé and Umbanda, during his doctorate in culture and society at the Federal University of Bahia (UFBA), when he studied the impact of hydroelectric dams on the São Francisco River on the ethnic groups of the backlands. In the Pankararé village of Brejo do Burgo, he met the shaman and chief Afonso Enéas, who taught him to collect black jurema and told him he was a son of Jurema, that one day he would work with it, but he did not feel a "driving effect" from the wine.

He experienced the takeoff with DMT from jurema combined with Syrian rue with the babalorixá, daimista, and juremeiro Reuber Rozendo, in Paulo Afonso (Bahia), where UNEB has a campus. He drank juremahuasca on the banks of the São Francisco and, under "a very strong impact," saw the spirits of the Indigenous people who had died in the region and the river transformed into a torrent of blood. "Spirits who spoke in Portuguese, that… impressed me. Outbreak, delirium, hallucination? It was then that I decided I would study these populations." He began drinking ayahuasca and jurema, but the latter prevailed: "It's a skin that adapts better to the ancestry of the sertão," the northeastern backlands. He became so fascinated that he decided to spread its use, holding rituals with university colleagues, in terreiros, and on the riverbank in Paulo Afonso.

With increasing land conflicts in the region, where people such as the Pankararé fought for recognition of their traditional areas occupied by farms, he was advised to leave the city and moved to Juazeiro, a municipality in Bahia neighboring Petrolina, on the opposite bank of the São Francisco river. There, he joined the movement against religious racism, responding to a call from the babalorixá Pai Jorge and Mãe Euzinha, who were accused of animal cruelty for sacrificing a goat.

He traveled through Europe, in Portugal and Spain, but upon returning to Brazil, his discomfort with psychoanalysis grew; he was not convinced by the description of mediumship as neurosis or psychosis. "It was easy [for a Lacanian] to accept medication and asylums, but not that a caboclo heals. And beating a little drum is free," he says, explaining his drift toward neo-shamanism. His pantheon now includes Pedro Luz, Yatra, and Rodrigo Grünewald, readings that convinced him of the usefulness of employing the Syrian rue inhibitor, which facilitates the effect of DMT in the brain. He found on his grandfather's land in the Serra dos Morgados "a quiet place to pray," but there he also encountered the threat of mining projects, joining the Salve as Serras (Save the Ranges) movement "to protect the sacred space of our mother."

Marques occupies the center of the Jurema egregore (collective spiritual force) he formed fifteen years ago with friends like Barreto, which almost dissolved during the covid-19 pandemic. He explains that the ceremonies are conducted under the guidance of three principles:

1. God is consciousness.
2. Nature is incarnate; the spiritual being must be incarnate.
3. The goal is to connect God with the deepest subjective consciousness of each individual.

"Our home is the Universe," he says. He is also responsible for preparing the juremahuasca and received the lyrics of many songs set to music by Edésio César, which everyone sings during their rituals,[9] such as "Juremeira":

There is a caboclo of Jurema
Mister Juremeira wears only feathers
Okê, okê, okê caboclo
Spin the world, Mister Juremeira
Bring in the rainbow of your plume
The power of the waterfall
I don't want gold
I don't want money
I just want straw
For my hut
I want to dance samba barefoot
In the yard of my village
Bring rain, feathered bird
For the harvest of mother jurema
Hail the power of Umbanda
Hail the lord of the mountains
Hail the Moon, hail the Sun
And the wolf that accompanies him

Several Deaths Under a Northeastern Golden Trumpet Tree and on Caymmi's Raft

After interviewing Juracy Marques, Claudia and I caught a ride with him to the Aldeia Pena Branca, the terreiro of his friend Pai João, who at 25 looks more like a university student than an Umbanda practitioner who has led the ceremonial house for six years, where we would drink juremahuasca. It was the first time that the group of Marques and Barreto gathered for this after the pandemic, in a ceremony organized to introduce the entheogen they produce and the song-centered ritual to the journalist from the Southeast. Together, they conduct the brief mandatory anamnesis interviews for those taking jurema for the first time, in order to minimize the risk of psychotic episodes or more serious physical problems (this is also common practice in ayahuasca religions; rarely does anyone serve the brew to people without knowing if they have a family history of psychosis or heart problems, if they take psychoactive medications, etc.). They recommend setting a clear intention before ingesting the drink and, in case of stronger disturbance, to take deep breaths and focus on the intention.

The space truly deserves the name terreiro (in Portuguese, a yard that has not been covered in tiles), for, between the street wall and the construction at the back with its altars, it features a space of about two hundred square meters of sand and many plants, among them a craibeira tree (*Tabebuia aurea*, also known as the ipê of caatinga). The ceremony takes place in this area, within a circle of white plastic chairs for about twenty people, with a few straw mats on the ground behind us. I receive the entheogen in half a disposable white plastic cup. The taste is unpleasant, a bitterness that unsettles the stomach. The sound system begins to play the 35 melodious and simple songs by César and Marques, ballads and marches that provide the guiding thread of the ritual, and I follow the lyrics for a while on a printed copy. I stop doing so when the force of the jurema comes on, overwhelming, and the words blur on the page.

I ask Claudia to call Marques or Barreto to help me as I leave the chair, and one of them assists me as I collapsed onto the mat beneath the craibeira. Lying down, the discomfort subsides, or I disconnect from it. I depart for an unknown place; later, in the sharing circle, I would say that I had died several times in those few hours. The sensation that I was about to dissolve is intense, but I always remain on that threshold, or at least I do not recall crossing it; perhaps the memory of the passage fades along with my dissolving consciousness or ego. But the absence is not complete, because I retain the memory of opening my arms and brushing them through the sand (later I would find my scalp full of it) when song number 20, "Ser sereno para a sereia" ("Be Serene for the Mermaid"), is sung:

> *Below I see the little shining dots*
> *Above I see the birds flying*
> *I enter your soul*
> *I reach the depths of the sea*
> *Odoiê, odoiá*
> *Yemanjá*

I open my eyes and see the iridescent craibeira, with an ethereal concreteness that lends it a certain personality, and I feel the tree making gestures toward me, as if on the verge of an embrace. The discomfort returns and I again ask for help to go to the bathroom, accompanied by Barreto. I try to vomit but cannot. The companion, who is a body therapist, asks permission to touch my waist, below the ribs, to see if he could unblock the vomiting, but there is nothing in my stomach, only an intense salivation. He then suggests we leave that place, which is not very conducive to spiritual experiences, and we laugh together. Back on the mat, the roller coaster starts again. Lyrics about Indigenous and African entities touch me viscerally; it is deeply unsettling. Barreto says the discomfort could be blocked mediumship. Sitting in the chair again, new waves of force give me the feeling that I could (should?) throw myself onto the sand, enter a trance, let it happen—what, exactly? Nothing happens, however.

I feel an excess of suffering in the world. The genocide and erasure of Black and Indigenous people is no joke, I conclude; it is not just victimhood, as right-leaning thinkers claim, it is something you can feel in your gut if you have the courage to look back and within. A young mixed-race woman speaks of violence in her family, and it disturbs me in a way that the intellectual cannot suppress. I don't say much in the sharing circle that follows, except to say that I have died several times and to thank everyone for the intense, in its own way beautiful, night. At one point I kneel on the sand and wrap my arms around Claudia's legs, laying my head in her lap like someone returning from a long journey and finally resting, or reciprocating—without any logic—the embrace I almost received from the craibeira. Once able to stand, I hug several people, including strangers.

It is up to Marques, once again, to take charge at the close of the gathering, which he does while embracing Pai João, the host, who says he had perhaps just experienced the most profound moment of his life, something he could only define by repeating a single word: "Love, love, love, love." But the professor from UNEB, at his side, does not feel comfortable in the role of guru, as he had pointed out in the afternoon interview: "They pressure me to become a pai de santo, a babalorixá. Everyone wants a master, but I don't believe in that role. Each person must take responsibility. I'm just another one trying to heal."

Rômulo Angélico, a catimbozeiro—as he prefers to define himself—from Natal, whom I met through Paulo de Azevedo, known as Purna, is less resistant to the role of spiritual leader. It was in a ritual led by him, on May 27, 2022, that I witnessed my first neo-shamanic ceremony using juremahuasca.[10]

I arrived by rideshare in the Redinha neighborhood of Natal, at the address provided by Mestre Rômulo, the same area of the Potiguar capital where, almost a century earlier, Mário de Andrade had undergone a spiritual protection ritual with Mestre Carlos. André Luiz, a nurse and the owner of the house, appeared on the street: "I don't live here, I hide here," he said, good-humoredly. I followed him down the alley from the ground down for fifty meters, up to the iron gate of the small house. "This house is no longer mine, it's yours now," he offered. In the small garden, he pointed to the right side as you enter, where a lit candle shone—the corner of Exu. There were already a few people in the living room, such as Mestre Breno, a young man named Iego, a woman from São Paulo, and two Argentine women, newcomers to jurema wine. Rômulo was sitting on the floor, beneath a painting of

Caboclo Pena Branca, the frame literally decorated with feathers ("penas" in Portuguese). On the same wall, there was a black-and-white picture of Jesus Christ; in the backyard, a cloth with the image of Ganesha, the elephant god of India. In front of the officiating master, a cardboard box with a laptop on top and objects such as pipes. The host indicated the spot in front of him for me to lay out my rubber mat. I took the snacks I had brought with me to the kitchen.

Mestre Rômulo gave an introductory talk for newcomers about what effects to expect from the three "doses" of Syrian rue and jurema we would take: we might have visions, vomit, and feel as if we were dying, but it would all pass and the cleansing would be beneficial. He dwelled a bit too long on the sensation of death, with support from Mestre Breno, who sounded more reassuring and declined Mestre Rômulo's invitation to officiate together: he said that the master in the room was Rômulo and that he greatly admired his courage in defending Catimbó. But Breno, who had been responsible for preparing the Syrian rue tea, did not miss the chance to give a lengthy explanation about the jurema flowers, which he smoked with a metal vaporizer that produced a sweet-smelling smoke. The next talk was about the traditional Tupinambá mantle made with scarlet ibis feathers, of which only a few examples remain today in European museums, one of them repatriated from Denmark in 2024, three centuries after being taken from Brazil. Mestre Breno took from his bag a kind of cap covered with blue macaw feathers, topped with a longer yellow one he called a "lightning rod," and a shawl painted with peacock feathers, composing something that for him represented that sacred mantle.

Mestre Breno offered the most beautiful metaphor of the night: after drinking the jurema, we would sail on a sea of ideas and fish. He wished everyone a good catch and sought to reassure us by saying that the boat had an owner, a captain, and a first mate, and that they would ensure everyone's safe return to solid ground. He then sang "Suíte do pescador" by Dorival Caymmi, though incomplete, focusing on the verses that speak of fishermen in a raft returning from the sea with a big catch, and thank God for the safe journey back, words that fit the night perfectly.

The session began around ten at night with the first chant led by Mestre Rômulo, who sang with a powerful, impressive bass voice. The lyrics spoke of Exu, masters, caboclos such as Pena Branca and Jurema, Our Lady, Saint Francis, and Saint Canindé. It must have been after eleven when we drank the first dose of Syrian rue; half an hour later, we took the jurema. In both cases, I asked to start with a small amount. I was surprised to feel something already with the rue alone, the onset of the characteristic tremor that psychedelics bring me, a shiver in my chest. The brownish tea made by Mestre Breno, with its peculiar vegetal taste, is taken before the jurema. The second drink is black and very bitter, and its preparation was Mestre Rômulo's responsibility. With the jurema itself, of which I also drank half a dose, I began to feel its effects in less than half an hour. Mestre Breno asked if I was all right and offered to complete the first dose, but I didn't feel the need. They sang a few more chants and then we listened to recorded music on the laptop connected to a small speaker. We were sitting on the floor, and soon I lay down.

Later I would describe the effect as very similar to ayahuasca, and at the same time very different. The first manifestations were visual: with my eyes closed, I began to see points and luminous spots that did not fill the entire space, as they would in a kaleidoscope. Soon they evolved into more complex, three-dimensional, architectural images: "Palaces of black glass and points of light," I wrote in my reporter's notebook. I think I also saw the thin face of a familiar woman, but I couldn't recognize her or retain the image for long. The visual part did not last long. Esoteric music (Andean, Indian, Native Brazilian) began to play to aid concentration. I dove into introspection, trying to direct it toward people like my brother and my father, but only women came to mind.

The "Prayer of Saint Francis" had played on the speaker, and perhaps because of that, the theme turned to forgiveness: I apologized to Monica for not having tried harder to write a story on the experimental breast cancer treatment she hoped to undergo in New York, and to my mother, Edith, for not being present at the time of her meningioma surgery, which put her in a coma due to an anesthetic accident and later killed her—a period when I was living in the United States. It was the most emotional moment, though not laden with guilt; nor was it exactly a request for forgiveness, more of a painful lament for not having provided the support that, I believe, would not have changed the course of the illnesses, but which they certainly would have appreciated. I also thought about my daughter Paula's illness, but without the anger, hurt, and revolt that usually accompany me—just a deep, calm sadness, of someone who accepts the world's suffering as it comes, though not with resignation; just sadness (when I recounted this, during the final round after the ritual was closed, my voice faltered).

I took the next dose, again in moderate quantity. After the second round, some people experienced incorporations of Jurema entities, such as Mestre Manoel Germano, the guiding spirt of Rômulo. The enchanted made his medium limp, put on a black hat, and smoked a pipe. Mestre Rômulo's torso jerked when an entity arrived or departed, but his voice did not change much, only his manner of speaking. I was neither impressed nor disturbed; I was not paying much attention to what was being said, absorbed in my own thoughts. André Luiz incorporated at least two entities, one of them a woman, possibly a pombajira. He put on a wide-brimmed hat adorned with a scarf, laughed a lot, loudly and theatrically. He walked around the room, passing among the seated and lying people, as if blessing them with his hands from a distance. He stopped by my side for quite a while, moving his hands back and forth. I am not sure how long this lasted, as I closed my eyes, almost indifferent to what was happening, but at some point the enchanted entity knelt beside me and asked permission to perform a healing. I replied, "Of course," sincerely and with mild curiosity, without apprehension.

She first touched my chest, moving back and forth until stopping over the upper right ribs. Her hand began to tremble in contact with my shirt, then the medium bent down and placed the mouth on the cloth, but I could not tell whether she was inhaling or blowing. I felt well, as if being caressed. Next, her hands moved down to my abdomen, where they trembled more. Somewhat agitated, almost shouting, she asked for a white candle, which she began to rub over my belly, stopping at a point where she broke it into three or four pieces still held together by the wick, which she threw away. She stood up without saying anything and resumed walking around the room.

I refused the third dose, as I was still under the effect and did not feel like continuing, and could well begin to come down. Chants and incorporations continued. Rômulo sang a União do Vegetal hymn about the Moon, which he said he found very beautiful and I found tedious. He played a song probably by Roberto Carlos, very long and religious, which I did not know. A young man sitting next to me seemed quite altered, after taking three doses of rue and jurema, using rape (snuff), and smoking a pipe in succession: he writhed sitting or standing, almost dancing, sometimes in strange positions, hissing loudly. In a less agitated moment, I took his hand and asked if he was all right. He smiled faintly and said yes.

Mestre Rômulo closed the ceremony and we sang together, now without a sound system, the third version of the "Prayer of Saint Francis," at the request of Mestre Breno, who referred to it as the "Chiquinho song" (he claimed it was not a Catholic Church hymn, but a song by an unknown author that Catholics had appropriated, "as they do with everything"). We then went to eat in the kitchen, while Mestre Rômulo delivered messages (advice from entities) in the living room to some of those present.

In the kitchen, André Luiz, the nurse and owner of the house, said he needed to talk to me about what had happened when the entity leaned over my body. He said he had felt a very strong aura around me, like a magnetic armor he could not penetrate, but that he needed to get through, which he insisted on and eventually managed. He said he associated what he felt in my lung with what I later said about sadness, because, "according to Chinese medicine," that is the seat of melancholy. He added that the bigger problem, however, was in the abdomen: he felt something very dark, a "knot of impurities" or something like that. He asked if I related this to anything, and at first I said no, that I had nothing in my abdomen, except that three years earlier I had undergone surgery to remove my prostate and its carcinoma, which tests indicated was cured. He said, "Ah, so that's it!".

He said he had felt the need to move his hand closer to my pubic area, but refrained from doing so to avoid seeming inappropriate or giving the wrong impression. I received the "confirmation" with my usual skepticism, since after all, everyone has something in their abdomen (diarrhea, cramps, nausea, heartburn, gas, liver, gallbladder, stomach problems, etc.), which makes it quite likely for a medium to detect something there, but I did not voice my disbelief. André Luiz then said, "Your healing was not three years ago, it was today. From now on, things will happen in your life."

(Less than two weeks after the "healing," I woke up at 4:30 a.m. tormented by diffuse pain that I initially attributed to intestinal cramps, perhaps a bout of diarrhea coming on. As it gradually worsened, without a single bowel movement, and began to concentrate on the left side, Claudia suspected it was a second episode of kidney stones and took me to the hospital. Bingo! I underwent stone removal by endoscopy and placement of a double J catheter, under general anesthesia. Before that, I even had morphine, twice, but the pain returned within minutes. I could not help but remember what André Luiz had told me. I asked Mestre Rômulo for his contact and wrote to him asking for the name of the entity that had incorporated at the moment he treated me. The integrative therapist with nursing training informed me that the entity had been the juremeira Mestra Ritinha.)

Master Rômulo came to ask how my experience had been, and I replied with something anodyne like "good, interesting" (and it truly was). I took the opportunity to ask who his guiding spirit was, and he told me a long story about how his godmother in the Jurema Sagrada, Maria Fernandes, had identified Manoel Germano, and how he gradually learned to receive and communicate with the enchanted being. But the most interesting story had happened years earlier, when he had not even considered Catimbó: he arrived at his aunt's house and found a twelve-year-old cousin wearing a hat, with a painted beard and mustache on her face, and dressed in a man's shirt. He thought she was in costume and asked why the girl had done that, to which she replied that there was no girl there, her name was Manoel Germano, and that he, Rômulo, would one day meet him.

In 2005, Rômulo was teaching history at a public school on the southern coast of Rio Grande do Norte. He knew little or nothing about Catimbó or Jurema Sagrada, barely distinguishing them from Candomblé or Umbanda. The local school system organized a science fair with the theme Religion in Canguaretama, and the students only came up with proposals on Christian topics. The future catimbozeiro master suggested Afro-Brazilian religions, and only fourteen out of 2,600 students showed any interest. From there, he delved deeper into the study of Northeastern religiosity, which led him to read works on Catimbó by Luís da Câmara Cascudo and Mário de Andrade. He also began visiting Indigenous communities and terreiros, where he interviewed catimbozeiros and took notes. In one of these conversations, he experienced what he calls "pre-mediumship," which he understood as a call to initiation.

From 2009 onward, he learned from shamans, juremeiro masters (including Breno and Maria Fernandes), and Umbanda practitioners (Francisca Bezerra Honorato, known as Neta from the Ogum-Odé terreiro) how to prepare jurema with water, honey, and wild varieties of cashew and passion fruit. In 2013, he opened his own terreiro, the Spiritualist Center House of the Rising Sun of King Malunguinho. The terreiro eventually closed after an act of vandalism, in which ritual objects were destroyed and pets were killed. "I do not perform [animal] sacrifices," Rômulo hastened to clarify. At the time of the ceremony in Redinha, he was working to open a new Catimbó space, the Spiritualist and Beneficent Center Master Manoel Germano—the neo-shamanic ritual I attended, for which he requested a contribution of eighty reais, was part of his fundraising efforts.

It was already past five in the morning and dawn was breaking. I grabbed my backpack and retrieved my phone, finding a message from Claudia at four asking where I was. I replied that I was having something to eat with the participants of the ceremony in Redinha and would soon call a rideshare. I was reluctant to be the first to leave, but I pulled myself together and asked permission to go. "Of course, brother, you are free to leave whenever you wish," replied Master Rômulo. I thanked him, requested the ride, and went to say goodbye to everyone individually. Master Breno only called me Psychonaut, because of the book, and I laughed. I left the house around 5:40, with an estimated time of arrival at 6:25. I had a long conversation with the driver, a 45-year-old former futsal player who had lived in São Paulo, Russia, and Croatia, brought there by the sport, but had never heard of jurema, ayahuasca, Catimbó, or Santo Daime. I received a rare compliment for being "very communicative" and arrived satisfied and happy at my hosts' house in Parnamirim, on the other side of the Natal metropolitan area.

I remain grateful to this day for the care Ritinha and André Luiz gave me that special night, under the effects of juremahuasca. On the other hand, just as the healing performed by them did not prevent the occurrence of a kidney stone crisis, neither my own journey propelled by DMT nor the spirit incorporations I witnessed led me to share the conviction in the existence of an enchanted realm where Ritinha, Manoel Germano, and Zé Pelintra reside. However, nor was it the case that I dismissed as pathological or pathetic the manifestations of those with whom I shared doses of entheogens, a snack, and several hours of ineffable joy among strangers—something incomprehensible under normal conditions. A few more steps in learning to accept the mystery as it presents itself, even when mixed in the postmodern blender of neo-shamanism, without feeling the need to lean on faith or doctrine to explain it.

Notes

1. The account of the Equinox festival is based largely on the report "Com ayahuasca e ioga, festival mistura psicodélicose rituais neoxamânicos," published in *Folha de S.Paulo* on April 7, 2022. Available at: https://www1.folha.uol.com.br/ilustrissima/2022/04/com-ayahuasca-e-ioga-festival-mistura-psicodelicos-e-rituais-neoxamanicos.shtml. Accessed: Dec. 31, 2024.
2. Graham St John, "Aussiewaska: a Cultural History of Changa and Ayahuasca Analogues in Australia", in Beatriz Caiuby Labate, Clancy Cavnar and Alex K. Gearin (Eds.), *The World Ayahuasca Diaspora: Reinvention and Controversies*. London/New York: Routledge, 2017. p. 156.
3. Jonathan Ott, "Psychonautic uses of 'Ayahuasca' and its Analogues: Panacæa or *Outré* Entertainment?" In: Beatriz Caiuby Labate, Henrik Jungaberle (Eds.). *The Internationalization of Ayahuasca*. Berlin: LIT Verlag, 2011. p. 109.
4. "Psychonautic uses of 'Ayahuasca' and its Analogues: Panacæa or *Outré* Entertainment?" In: Beatriz Caiuby Labate, Henrik Jungaberle (Eds.). *The Internationalization of Ayahuasca*. Berlin: lit Verlag, 2011. p. 120.
5. "Aussiewaska: a Cultural History of Changa and Ayahuasca Analogues in Australia", in Beatriz Caiuby Labate, Clancy Cavnar and Alex K. Gearin (Eds.), *The World Ayahuasca Diaspora: Reinvention and Controversies*. London/New York: Routledge, 2017.

6. Graham St John, "Aussiewaska: a Cultural History of Changa and Ayahuasca Analogues in Australia", p. 155.

7. Esther Jean Langdon, "New Perspectives of Shamanism in Brazil". *Civilisations*, v. 61, n. 2, pp. 30–1, 28 Jun. 2013.

8. * Disintrusion refers to the removal from indigenous lands of residents and squatters who settled there after the beginning of the identification process of the traditional territory.

9. Available at: https://open.spotify.com/playlist/0hWBRfIV7xD25Ho T1DxWXS?si=5ja3Ej5OT9u0MvD2hDJfoA&pi=u-GFiM_t6qSJm2. Accessed on: 20 Dec. 2024.

10. Ceremony partially narrated in the report "Cultos com alucinógeno da jurema florescem no Nordeste," published in *Folha de S.Paulo* on July 26, 2022. Available at: https://www1.folha.uol.com.br/ilustrissima/ 2022/07/cultos-com-alucinogeno-da-jurema-florescem-no-nordeste. shtml. Accessed on: 20 Dec. 2024.

The Eternal Return of Mysticism

On November 15, 2022, I discovered that journalistic detachment can end up at your feet. I was attending the baptism of seven juremeiros at the Tenda de Umbanda Caboclo Pena Branca and Casa de Catimbó Mestre Junqueiro, in the Santo André neighborhood of Belo Horizonte (capital city of the state of Minas Gerais, in the Southeast of Brazil), when I realized I was the only one wearing shoes and socks among about thirty people. Everyone else was barefoot, as is tradition in many terreiros, but I decided to remain as I had entered, without direct contact with the beige porcelain floor that the initiates had diligently cleaned hours earlier. The camera for taking photos and videos, as well as the notebook, already imposed enough distance; there was no reason to simulate an adherence that did not actually exist. "Objectivity," I wrote in my notebook, with somewhat ironic quotation marks, driven by my usual skepticism regarding spirituality.

The path to Pai Orestes' terreiro had been winding. I had met him three months earlier at an ayahuasca ceremony at the Instituto Nhanderu, in the "cracolândia" (crackland) area of downtown São Paulo, as a guest of Adriano de Camargo and Sebastiana da Silva Fontes, known as Tuca, who work with drug addicts and the homeless in that degraded part of the city. The couple knew that this book on jurema was in preparation and introduced me to Orestes as a consecrated juremeiro working outside the Northeast where black jurema grows, which fit my thesis that the cult of Jurema Sagrada was expanding beyond its region of origin (although I did not have then, nor do I have now, statistical data to back this). We exchanged several messages until we settled on the Republic Day holiday, when a baptism ceremony would

M. Leite, *The Psychedelic Science of the Jurema Tree*, Copernicus Books, https://doi.org/10.1007/978-3-032-22705-8_7

take place, as the most suitable date to witness a complete ritual—in fact, two: baptism in the morning and jurema de chão in the afternoon.

When I arrive at the terreiro at 9:15 a.m., the house members are already busy cleaning the large hall with buckets of water and soap, mops, and a hose, in an almost childlike festive atmosphere. Along the wall facing the entrance, there is a table covered with a white cloth, on which a myriad of Jurema ceremonial objects can be seen, such as maracás, glasses of water, keys, pipes, candles, bells, and images of sacred entities. In the left corner, a green seven-pointed cross and a coat rack with a collection of hats. The back wall is painted blue and has several glass shelves with groups of images: malandros (notably Zé Pelintra), pretos velhos, orixás, saints, and gypsies on the lower part; higher up, Santa Bárbara (syncretized as Iansã) and São Jerônimo (Xangô); at the very top, above all, Jesus Christ (Oxalá), highlighted by a powerful spotlight. At the other end of the hall, there is a room that serves as an office and a small shop for ceremonial objects, such as pipes and statuettes, as well as the doors to the bathroom and kitchen.

After the cleaning, disciples set up a mat in the center of the room, covered with leaves and herbs. There are also white flowers and clay dishes with apples, tangerines, mangoes, melons, watermelons, coconuts, papayas, bananas, oranges, grapes, and pineapples. A large blue plastic basin filled with water is placed in the center, and the soon-to-be baptized begin adding herbs to it, preparing the scented water: jasmine, basil, lavender, boldo, pitanga, rosemary, and guiné. Seated in a circle, they echo Jurema chants led by a woman in a yellow turban, who circles the group puffing on a rustic pipe. At 10:45 a.m., Orestes, wearing gray shorts and an orange t-shirt, a white hat on his head, joins them. He seems agitated, using rapé (snuff) and blowing clouds of smoke from the pipe, and enters the circle ringing a bell over the basin of herbal bath. He leads several prayers: the Lord's Prayer, Hail Mary, Hail Holy Queen, and the Guardian Angel prayer. He invokes the caboclos and sings: "Go seek Science in that deep basement." He gives instructions on how to arrange the hall for the baptism ritual proper, which will follow.

Everyone returns dressed in white, including Orestes. A young woman sits separated from those who will be baptized, on a mat covered with a white sheet under the window to the left of the blue altar wall, where she will remain all day, withdrawn in preparation to assume more prominent ritual functions in the house. In front of her, dishes with "foods of the earth," as Orestes explains: honey, yam, pumpkin, and cassava. This is the caboclo's mat, where the initiate remains in contact with the ground before the offerings, among them the jurema wine, which gives the caboclos—entities that were once Indigenous persons—wisdom and strength for hunting. The purpose of this isolation is to give the young woman "the energy of the pajé, of the warrior," the house leader explains, so she can "enter this energetic and spiritual form: strength, balance, and tranquility."

Her name is Luzinete Roscoe Correa Pinto, she is 33 years old and teaches English and Spanish at a private high school in Belo Horizonte. Raised Catholic, she knew nothing of Umbanda or Jurema Sagrada when she was brought to the terreiro in 2018 by her boyfriend, now her husband. At first, she only helped out at the small shop and organized the line of people waiting to consult with Pai Orestes. Over time, as she immersed herself in the rituals, she began to understand the symbols, and two years later, she discovered the name of her own caboclo: "We all have our entities; it's a matter of developing them. It's not an easy path."

In addition to the classes she teaches, she works at her brother's travel agency. She lived for a month in Ireland and another in Argentina to improve the languages she studied in the language and translation courses at the Federal University of Minas Gerais. She has been postponing the plan to have children because "in today's Brazil it's complicated," and lives with her husband and seven cats, animals that Orestes, by her side, explains are symbols of magic, strength, and cunning. The main challenge in her religious path lies in what she calls political issues, the frequent attacks on terreiros, and the barriers that must be overcome to freely express her faith. At the school where she works, she did not initially disclose her religion, fearing that the adolescents, who are very anxious, would not react well. Over time, she gained confidence and began to wear her guides (beaded necklaces), which aroused the curiosity and questions of the students. She then told them about the Native and Afro-Brazilian religion's social initiatives, such as distributing food and toys to the poor. She also had no issues with her fellow teachers, as some of them were Kardecist spiritists. She is taking a degree course in English to improve her position in the job market and attends the terreiro every Wednesday and Friday.

> *Let us honor the masters of Jurema*
> *Let us honor Solomon*
> *Let us honor Jurema*
> *For it is our duty*
> *In the forest there is a caboclo*
> *All dressed in feathers*
> *His name is Malunguinho*
> *Do not meddle with him*
> All translations of lyrics, verses and quotes from Portuguese to English are the author's with help of AI

The chants that Orestes sings in front of Luzinete, amid the puffs of smoke, seem to have an effect on the young woman (all translations of quotes, verses and lyrics from Portuguese are the author's with help of AI). Seated, she leans back and forth, at times touching her forehead to the mat. She twists her hands, one arm in her lap and the other behind her back, breathing deeply. Her movements intensify, her arms now outstretched, touching the white cloth with her index fingers pointed. My heart starts to beat faster and I jot down in my notebook: "There is something in the air beyond the smoke." After forty minutes of singing and smoke, Orestes tells her she can let the caboclos come under the power of the maracás during the baptism that is about to begin, but she must not leave the mat: "The connection is yours." Thunder rumbles.

Orestes then begins a lecture for the future initiates, seated on small benches with hats, candles, jurema wood pipes, maracás, and goblets with necklaces of gray and white beads known as Our Lady's tears in front of them. He says they must ask permission to enter Jurema and tread carefully on another's land: "Everything is responsibility." He instructs them to begin the fumigation, and a young man in a floral shirt walk around the hall with a censer, wafting smoke over each attendee. The woman in the yellow turban moves around with her left hand behind her back, thumb and forefinger pointed like an arrow, kneels twice, taps her chest with the maracá, extends it toward the initiates, and, as she passes me, touches my left shoulder with it. New invocations to Jurema and Solomon are sung.

The baptism itself begins. Orestes stands in front of each initiate and pours herbal water over their heads. He takes the beaded cord from the goblet, washes it, and ties it around the initiate's neck, then hands them the goblet and the pipe. He returns to the start of the line and blows smoke into the goblets filled with jurema wine, which the disciple then drinks. Everyone sings: "Jurema is an enchanted wood/A wood of knowledge/That everyone wants to know." The master of Jurema walks down the line again and kisses the hands of each young person as they repeat: "I was baptized in the law of God, my godfather and godmother were assigned to me by God." He gives them the hat to place on their heads, "the sorcerer's protection," Orestes explains, announcing a Jurema de Chão ritual for after lunch.

The second ceremony begins around 3:30 p.m. with several prayers: the Lord's Prayer, Hail Mary, Hail Holy Queen, Saint John of the Lord, Saint Anthony… They sing:

With his leather jacket
His crown of thorns
Oh arrow, arrow I

Kings Malunguinho

An hour later, I begin to yawn uncontrollably, as if about to enter the force after drinking ayahuasca or juremahuasca, but that is not the case. With my eyes closed, listening to the singing and the continuous sound of the maracás, I concretely understand the importance attributed by the psychologist and psychedelic guru Timothy Leary to *setting* (environment), alongside *set* (mental disposition) and substance, to define the quality of the psychedelic experience: even without ingesting any entheogen, one feels the approach of a threshold of consciousness triggered by the ritual, resembling the transition from wakefulness to sleep, as if a hypnotic effect were added to the smoke and its penetrating odor. The effect has something to do with sensory saturation, as if the strong rhythm and singing overpower one's control, the filter that allows us to make rational sense of things in this world.

Orestes, who like almost all the initiated men now wears a colorful chintz shirt and a hat, rolls up the cuffs of his white pants. The young woman sitting to my right, with red hair and a lace skirt with golden stripes worn over burgundy pants, stretches out to the floor and tenses her index fingers and thumbs, trembling. A thin young man beats his chest with crossed arms, a wooden arrow in each hand. A bald man in a straw hat drinks cachaça and spits a jet onto the feet of the woman in burgundy pants, who has already discarded her skirt, apparently embodying another entity. I count at least seven people in trance. The tall bearded man who had given me a plate of food now walks around the hall with a cane and black hat, smoking a pipe and singing:

> *My God, what city is that*
> *That I see from afar?*
> *I am Tertuliano*
> *Resident of Afogados*
> *On the right I am gentle*
> *On the left I am heavy*

He comes over to talk to me and asks if I came from far away—yes. He says that the spirits are pleased with my presence and mumbles something about finding the path by listening to the heart. He grabs my hand with his and beats both against my chest. I get goosebumps and reply that I was learning. Next, it is Orestes who manifests, dominating the hall with a shrill laugh, crooked staff in one hand and a glass of cachaça in the other, embodying Mestre Pé de Garrafa. A line forms in front of him for blessings, and the most beautiful woman comes to ask if I want to go speak with him—I reply no, and it is at that exact moment that I realize I am the only one wearing socks and shoes.

Orestes drinks several times from the bottle and does the same with the initiates, particularly with a young man to whom he serves repeated doses, until the young man finally musters the courage to refuse and puts an end to the entity's test, to everyone's laughter. The padrinho sits down and asks for the maracá. He hisses, sighs, and moans, showing signs that he is disembodying his master. He intones: "O God, bless the holy chalice and the consecrated host." Some women begin to receive the spirits of cowboys, shouting "êêê boi!", making gestures as if throwing lassos to capture "any negative energy left in the house" and striking the floor hard with a whip. It is almost 7:30 p.m. when Orestes goes from person to person giving hugs. To me, he wishes "much strength for your family and your journey," then asks if I can drive the golden Corolla, a gift from a goddaughter, to his house. The lights come on, and everyone laughs at José, who keeps singing chants, alone, inside the bathroom.

Orestes Mineiro de Sousa Junior was fifty years old when I interviewed him the next day, in his apartment in the Planalto neighborhood of Belo Horizonte, the city where he was born into a family of merchants. His grandfather, Jorge Saad, had been the Syrian consul in the state capital. His mother, an educator, was the one who led him and his brother to the "spiritual path" in a theosophical organization, the Great White Brotherhood, where a select few had access to the teachings of Ascended Masters, among whom was said to be Jesus Christ himself. Even before attending law school, which he would do at the age of thirty, at nineteen he first dedicated himself to the study of occultism and hermeticism in the Order of the Templars of Belo Horizonte, being initiated at twenty-four as a master mason. In a "difficult phase of life," his first wife took him for consultations at an Umbanda house, the Cabana de Caridade São Francisco de Assis, run by Mãe Ruth. Under the scent of incense during the rituals, his body would tremble and he experienced tachycardia, but he did not like what would be the first signs of mediumship. After two years attending the terreiro, in 2006, a guide, Pai Benedito, told him he needed to work on it, upon seeing Orestes start to jump on the bench as soon as Mãe Ruth placed a rosary around his neck.

With his path set, he began the "relentless search" that would lead him to open his own house in 2016. He was initiated into Quimbanda, an Afro-Brazilian religious tradition with an emphasis on magic and the worship of exus and pombajiras. He discovered the Jurema Sagrada in São Paulo and received a message from Caboclo Pena Branca that he should seek it at its source, in the Northeast. In 2015, he traveled to Paraíba, where he met with Pajé Antônio, of the Potiguara people, in Baía da Traição, with Pai Beto de Xangô, in João Pessoa, and with Lucas, grandson of Mestra Jardecilha, in

Alhandra. The meeting was scheduled with Nina, Lucas's mother, but Orestes lost the address; he only knew she lived near the school. When he stopped the car in front of the school, a young man with a hat and pipe came out of a house saying he had been waiting for him—it was Lucas. He had scheduled a half-hour conversation and remained three, next to the "cities" (trees) of jurema that the family struggles to keep alive in the backyard. In 2019, he would return to the Paraiban mecca of Jurema Sagrada to undergo the "tombamento," a ritual practiced in some houses that corresponds to the highest degree of initiation for a juremeiro—a kind of official recognition as a priest, authorizing him to have godchildren and baptize initiates, after visiting Tambaba beach and asking for permission. The person literally collapses after drinking the wine, he recounts: "You black out, it's not like ayahuasca, where you remain awake. Both the drink and the ritual act guide you. It's strange, you're focused, singing, then you hear a name in your head and start to feel mental, emotional, and physical sensations—there's a certainty that it's your spirit speaking."

There are several entities that Orestes receives, from Umbanda, Quimbanda, and Jurema Sagrada, whose rituals he keeps on separate days, despite the fine line that separates them, in his view. In Quimbanda, Exu Marabô, honored with a tattoo on his left wrist; on the right wrist, a Zé Pelintra hat and a Maria Padilha rose, who appear in both Umbanda and Jurema. But there is also room, in his mediumship, for caboclos and masters such as Pena Branca, Junqueiro, Pé de Garrafa, and Júlia Galega. Jurema is everything to him today: "Umbanda is my mother, but Jurema is my grandmother. My fortress, my foundation, along with Quimbanda." Umbanda has become somewhat stagnant, he says, too commercialized. In his experience, people crave something more closed, more mysterious, and Jurema appeals to that curiosity.

Stepping outside the Quadrant in a São Paulo Jurema House

After two years traveling to learn about the power of DMT from black jurema and some of the many manifestations of Jurema Sagrada throughout Brazil, particularly among Indigenous people, spiritual leaders, and neo-shamans of the Northeast, I finally succeed in making contact with the nearest terreiro: Espaço Jurema Mestra, in Santo André, in the metropolitan region of São Paulo, my home town. The place was opened in 1990 by Paulo Alcântara, a juremeiro from Recife, who welcomes my partner Claudia and me to the

Festa das Mestras with an apology for the delay in responding to messages. He points to white plastic chairs for visitors to sit on, at the entrance, in the narrowest part of the hall. He asks if I am from Umbanda or Candomblé, to know how to address me, and I reply that I am from neither. As he shakes our hands, he apologizes again, this time for his long fingernails painted green: "Don't be surprised, it's because of the entity I receive." He wears a short-brimmed black hat, dark pants, a yellow shirt, and a necklace of green and white glass beads.

We are on the third and top floor of a small building above a bar, in front of the Cristo Operário church, a rooftop covered with a fiber cement roof that widens ahead into what Alcântara calls the Quadrant. He explains that he will soon call us to witness, up close, the ritual of that December 3, 2023. It is the area reserved for initiates, many women in turbans and men in hats sitting on black plastic stools around the perimeter of the square marked on the floor, with a six-pointed star in the center. The loft is open on the left side, without windows, and the back wall is covered with pink and beige curtains, in front of which, on the floor, is a profusion of bowls with fruit and flowers. In the center of the Quadrant, a small table serves as an altar for Our Lady of the Conception, with two candlesticks holding lit candles and a rosary of giant beads at her feet. To the right, a wall filled with objects: gourds, maracás, straw hats, portraits of Catholic saints.

The owner of the terreiro begins a lecture on the Sacred Jurema, the religion of the ancestors for whom they will pray the rosary: "Jurema is a cultural puzzle. Sometimes it's hard to understand," he warns. He says that Jurema was already present in São Paulo, but conditioned by Umbanda, and that he himself was a pioneer in presenting it as it is, with its own rituals and cosmogony, with its maracás and ilus (drums). He tells a bit of the history of Catimbó in the Northeast, how it gained fame in the city of Alhandra with Mestra Maria do Acais, and how he had to face "backward concepts," striking the statue of Padre Cícero with his left hand, in reference to the Catholic Church. One of Acais's initiates was Maria Dagmar, he says, who became known as Joana Pé de Chita and initiated another woman, Joana de Santa Rita, who in turn initiated Dona Nilza, Alcântara's mother and mentor in Jurema. "She didn't leave me money, but she left me knowledge."

By around five in the afternoon, there are at least sixty people, both visitors and initiates, when the master rings the bell to begin the rosary, which will be dedicated to Our Lady of the Conception, "godmother of the sixteen kingdoms of Jurema." He orders the candles to be lit. "Praised be Our Lord Jesus Christ. Who is greater than God?" Everyone responds: "No one." Then they repeat the first four verses of a Catholic prayer ten times:

Mary goes ahead
And opens the paths
Opening doors and gates
Opening homes and hearts

Each person receives a candle with a blue ribbon to light from the flame already burning beside the image of Our Lady of the Immaculate Conception and to make a wish. The group recites an Our Father and a Hail Mary, extinguishes the flames, and the untied ribbons, placed in a glass urn, will be taken by Alcântara to Recife. This is followed by a photo and selfie session beside the Virgin. The master moves around, sprinkling water with jurema over those present. Two songs are sung for Malunguinho, who is offered a bowl of fruit and a bottle of cachaça. The jurema wine, whose recipe Alcântara keeps secret, is served from a large bottle only to those within the Quadrant.

A newly initiated young man, Eduardo, ascends the stairs guided by Kaike, Alcântara's right-hand man in the terreiro. He enters wearing a feathered headdress and white clothing, along with a small wooden bow and arrow that looks like a toy in his hands, embodying the spirit Caboclo Pena Branca. The chief juremeiro blows copious pipe smoke over the young initiate, who dances on the star drawn on the floor to the sound of the ilus painted with yellow and white stripes. His appearances will be repeated throughout the ceremony, each time with different entities characterized by their attire, such as a strapless dress. Several other men do the same: descending the stairs and returning incorporated as Jurema mistresses to whom the night is dedicated, speaking and laughing loudly, smoking heavily, asking for wine or beer under the watchful eye of Alcântara, who constantly reminds everyone that alcoholic beverages are intended only for the entities.

The celebration continues for a long time. Around eight o'clock, Claudia and I decide to leave, despite Alcântara's protests, who promises a "little snack" soon and the incorporation of his own mistress, Cigana Rosa—something we will only witness weeks later in a social media video, as we stick to our decision to leave the ritual. The juremeiro expresses deep gratitude for our presence.

Before leaving, a woman who had been by my side for almost the entire time on the periphery of the quadrant hugs me tightly and, with a hoarse voice and piercing, slightly unsettling gaze, asks permission to tell me something: "You have little faith, that's why it takes you so long to get what you're seeking," she whispers, making gestures indicating that I grasp things with one hand and let them slip away with the other, for lack of belief. This time I was barefoot, in respect for the customs of the place, and had no camera, only my notebook. Yet, even so, the reporter's detachment did not go unnoticed by the perceptive entity who embraced me.

Years of Pilgrimage in Search of a Registration for a One-Person Psychedelic Church

Mark Ian Collins, an unlikely Anglo-Brazilian juremeiro who had spent thirteen years trying to open a church devoted to DMT, picked me up at Fortaleza airport that Friday, March 10, 2023. From there, we drove to the home of psychologist and indigenous rights advocate Luiz Lacerda Sousa Cruz, who had organized our trip to Caucaia, in the metropolitan area of Ceará's capital, where we would take part in a jurema ceremony. The gathering would be held in an area belonging to the Tapeba Indigenous people, who reemerged—or regained recognition—in the 1980s as the inhabitants of the Nossa Senhora dos Prazeres de Caucaia village, which in fact gave its name to the municipality.[1]

It is half past nine at night when we arrive in two cars at the home of Mestra Margarida by the Tapeba lagoon. Beyond the backyard is a sandy terreiro around a white jurema tree, where the hostess and Maria Salete Pessoa Guimarães, both dressed in white, await us. As we talk about the eito fishing technique, in which curimatás, traíras, cangatis, pirambebas, and even pitus (freshwater shrimp) are corralled in the lagoon, Salete lights a pipe and Mark pulls his from the shoulder bag he carries. We sing happy birthday to Margarida, who is celebrating, and the mistress announces that there is ayahuasca, jurema wine, and rapé to be taken. There are eleven of us in the terreiro: some take rapé, others daime, but Mark and I opt for jurema, served in disposable plastic coffee cups. As is common in the preparation of the wine by indigenous peoples, it has a sweet flavor and a subtle effect, which few would describe as psychedelic. Margarida gives each person a white candle to pray to their guardian angel and then place at the base of the jurema tree.

A nephew of Margarida is about to drink jurema for the first time, which prompts Mark to launch into a speech about the young man's privilege, comparing his early initiation to his own, as he only drank the northeastern entheogen at age 48 (he had known ayahuasca since he was 21, but it had little impact on his life). This is followed by a toré, circling the tree full of candles lit for the angels, with the women singing various Jurema chants in a relaxed ritual. Margarida wears a tall feathered headdress and, after the dance, walks back and forth on the sand around the bonfires, letting out a few hisses and gesturing with her arms. It is nearly two in the morning when roasted fish and sweet potatoes are served; I eat little. At the back of the property is a wattle-and-daub hut dedicated to the pretos velhos (African ancestors), where a few hammocks are strung. Exhausted, I settle into one, dozing more than sleeping to the sound of continuous conversation and from the buzzing of mosquitoes, I only got up to eat a bit of sausage I'd heard about amid the stupor.

Lacerda calls Mark and me to go to the edge of the lagoon, about twenty meters beyond the pretos velhos hut. It's the magical moment of the night: under the full moon, the leaves of the mangrove trees shine with silvery tones, as if I were seeing, for the first time, a plant intentionally emitting its own light. We sit there on the bank for a few enchanting minutes. Back at the yard, close to dawn, the indigenist asks what I learned about Cabocla Jurema; when I answer, using the expression "Indigenous religiosity," Margarida immediately reacts, explaining that Indigenous peoples do not have religion, but spirituality (and Lacerda adds: the Tapeba had very traumatic experiences with the religion imposed by the colonizer). I return to the silence I had maintained throughout the night, somewhat detached from the ceremony. Lacerda heads back to Fortaleza to care for his recently operated wife. Mark and I stay to share coffee brewed right there, over the embers of the dying fire.

Mark was born in Rio de Janeiro to a Brazilian mother, Marise Botelho Collins, and an English father, Colin Peter Collins, a technician who worked at the Western Telegraph Co. branch in the state of Maranhão, where he installed submarine cables.[2] The foreigner went to celebrate Carnival in Fortaleza, Ceará, and, during the festivities, met his future wife, a young woman recently returned from an exchange program in the United States and the only one in the hall who spoke English. When Mark was two years old, the family moved to England and then to Bermuda—but he stayed behind, at eight years old, studying at Barrow Hills boarding school in Willey, Surrey. There were only about a hundred students at the school, and the boy's only amusement was the library, where he became fascinated by the lives of the saints. He returned to live in Fortaleza at thirteen, when his father left the Cable & Wireless subsidiary for good to make a life in Brazil, settling in his wife's hometown. Mark ended up at another Catholic school, Colégio Santo Inácio.

His spiritual readings continued in the library of his grandfather from Ceará, a theosophy enthusiast. His curiosity was piqued by Brazil's eclectic religious landscape, and he immersed himself in terreiros and esoteric groups dedicated to astrology, occultism, and alchemy, becoming a professional astrologer in the 1980s. He hosted the radio program *Moon Tips* on

Jangadeiro radio station, an almanac in which he discussed the calendar and made comments for each zodiac sign, but without the predictions that would characterize a horoscope. "It was all very technical," he says. His first contact with ayahuasca was at age 21, but he only began regular use at 29, when he joined the church União do Vegetal (UDV).

In the meantime, he got married, had two children, got divorced, worked at the former airline Transbrasil, and studied philosophy and mechanical engineering, without graduating. Shortly after, he moved to Minas Gerais with plans to live a simple life on a small farm, after remarrying. With his money frozen by the Collor Plan in 1990, he was unable to buy property and worked as an astrologer in an office next to the sauna at the Palace Hotel in Caxambu (Minas Gerais). At that time, he discovered the Figueira farm, founded by José Trigueirinho Netto (1931–2018) from São Paulo, a kind of alternative monastery now known as the Figueira Community of Light, where he lived for a year. He returned to Fortaleza in 1995 at his mother's request, who was raising Mark's two children, and worked in electronic publishing. At an esoteric retreat in the Aratuba mountains, he met Maria das Graças, a pharmacist, whom he married and has been with for three decades. She convinced him to finish at least one university degree (theology), and since then has supported him in his life project: the Church of the Divine Master on Earth (IDMT, as in Portuguese acronym).

It was in mid-2008, during his master's in philosophy on the concept of utopia in Thomas More, that Mark began his independent shamanic work. He took the opportunity to buy two liters of ayahuasca through a member of the Barquinha church, just as his wife was leaving for three months of training in Canada, and stored the bottle on top of the bookshelf, wrapped in aluminum foil, not really knowing what to do with the entheogen. After hearing about the psychedelic effects of jurema, he called a cousin in Pacatuba, in the metropolitan region of Fortaleza, where he knew there were patches of caatinga, to order black jurema roots. The relative hired three young men for the job, who, curious about the plant's psychoactivity, made a tea with it that only caused them to vomit. Upon receiving payment for the task, Mark says, they went to drink cachaça but couldn't, their stomachs turning at the smell of the liquor; then they tried to smoke crack, also without success.

Mark says that when he heard this story over the phone, his knees shook. He then asked his cousin to see if the young men wanted to try "a real lombra," Brazilian slang for the buzz or effect of psychoactive drugs—and they agreed. Off went the philosopher with his two liters of ayahuasca for a session at the small farm by the Quiobal reservoir. After a full cup of the brew, they found the effect marvelous: "They burst into adjectives, trying to explain the ineffable," Mark recalls. "They got exactly where I wanted them to go." They asked if there would be new meeting the following week, and they began bringing friends to the sessions, which led to rumors spreading that miracles were being performed at Quiobal with drug addicts who were giving up drugs.

In this informal setting, the Anglo-Brazilian discovered what he still considers his calling: to provide others with the beatific experiences he himself had with ayahuasca, and smoked DMT crystals (changa), which had changed his life for the better. To try to do this legally, he conceived the idea of founding a neo-shamanic congregation around this sacrament, the IDMT. The same acronym also refers to two other organizations included in the project: the Institute of the Tryptamine Molecule (focused on education) and the Institute of Multidisciplinary Therapeutics (to promote participants' well-being)—as well as the emblem of his vocation, which he sums up in the English expression "*IDMT*."

The eccentricity of the IDMT lies in the fact that it proposes itself as a one-member church—its founder, Mark Ian Collins. Anyone else who attends is merely a participant, not a member, and may retain their own beliefs and previous affiliations. Even atheists are welcome, to counterbalance the discrimination against them in Brazilian law, which only allows the legal use of an entheogen containing DMT (in this case, ayahuasca) in a ritual context. The religious reference for the IDMT is Jurema Sagrada, heir to Catimbó, a fluid set of magical-spiritual practices from the Northeast backlands centered on the consumption of jurema wine. The bible of the nascent IDMT is the bilingual book *The Path of a Juremeiro*,[3] written in three days, according to Mark. It contains 238 stanzas of seven rhymed lines in Portuguese, imitating cordel literature to honor Northeastern culture, with a free English translation on each facing page. The work reads:

> *The need for a new belief*
> *is that it does not fit into something that already exists.*
> *that would greatly limit its scope*
> *something that I consider unwise.*
> *So I come with this novelty*
> *without any pomposity or vanity*
> *of wanting to build a different church*

And also, highlighting the parallel that Mark sees between Northeastern religiosity and the Amazonian ayahuasca, or daime, cult and its power plants mariri and chacruna, the latter called the Queen:

> *Hail to the Indian woman Jurema*
> *who is the Queen of the Sertão,*
> *just as the Queen of the Forest*
> *who is our Lady of Conception*
> *Jurema is Our Lady of Graces*
> *that fills our glasses,*
> *to consecrate our religion.*

The plan to officially open and register the one-member church with the molecule as its sacrament proved to be a quixotic endeavor. Once the idea emerged, in 2011, Mark dedicated himself to drafting the bylaws, later rendered in verse, consulted lawyer Felipe Trazzi Carvalho, and went to the notary's office with the founding act drawn up at the Lagoinha farm in Paracuru (Ceará), a coastal municipality in the metropolitan region of Fortaleza (the planned headquarters was never established). According to paragraph 4 of article 2 of the bylaws, the IDMT would be configured as "a place for vertical relationship, connecting the participant with themselves, the spiritual world, and the Divine." In article 4, the purpose of the church is defined as "study, research, and shamanic religious practice." However, the notary official forwarded the registration request to the courts with a "statement of doubt" regarding the legality of a religious association of that kind. In an attempt to challenge the notary's decision, Mark and the lawyer wrote to the judge in March 2014:

> Today, there are movements both among Indigenous peoples and within academia to revive and rediscover this religious culture, which is the only one that can be described as 100% Brazilian, as it did not receive any external influence in its development—only in its destruction. (Author's translation with the help of artificial intelligence)

Upon consultation, the State Attorney Office of Ceará opined in July 2014 that the IDMT sought to employ lawful means (religious) to achieve unlawful ends (obtaining ayahuasca for purposes beyond the religious). Prosecutor Elizabela Rebouças Tomé Praciano also objected to the notion of a single-member church and required that the National Health Surveillance Agency (ANVISA) also be heard, since the IDMT intended to conduct study and research with a controlled substance. In December of the same year, the petitioner submitted another objection, arguing that the study and research aimed to establish safe dosages and provide transparency to participants in the ceremonies. Mark Collins was subjecting his belief to scientific scrutiny in order to show that what was previously witnessed, presumably under the effect of the entheogen, is not merely an illusion, the petition argued. The Divine reveals itself both to the scientist and to the mystic, it went on. "It is incomprehensible how the distinguished representative of the Attorney's Office can claim that study and research do not constitute a religious practice."

In May 2015, Judge Francisco Marcelo Alves Nobre ruled that the registration of the IDMT could be processed by the notary office under one condition: that Anvisa authorize the use of DMT. When contacted, the agency responded that it was only authorized to grant permission to companies. In July, Mark petitioned that, by exclusion, Anvisa could not regulate religious organizations, and in September, that the plant black jurema, like the chacruna and mariri of ayahuasca (the three sources of psychedelics listed by his church for ceremonial use), did not fall under the agency's jurisdiction. In July of the following year, 2016, the Ceará Attorney's Office stated it no longer opposed the organization's registration, and in September, Judge Wyrllenson Flávio Barbosa Soares authorized it.

Eight years later, as the manuscript of this book was being finalized, no official function of the IDMT had yet taken place. Experimental sessions with the entheogen occurred until the onset of the covid-19 pandemic in 2020, which interrupted the process of establishing a physical headquarters in Fortaleza and transferring the registration address. It was only in November 2023 that the project was fully formalized in the capital of Ceará, ten years after the bylaws and *The Path of a Juremeiro* were drafted, but with its registered office in a coworking space and always on the verge of beginning sessions. Mark uses a distinctly Brazilian metaphor to describe the current stage of his church: "The IDMT Project is being born in the taxi, the water has already broken, the head is already out, crying, general panic, but it's being born, it seems it can no longer be contained, as it was for so long by my fears and insecurities," he said in a message. "The creature has awakened and even without being fully 'delivered'—that is, even without being inaugurated—things are already happening."

A Veil of Science over Perennialism Resurrected by the Power of DMT

The doctrine of the IDMT involves a peculiar blend of neo-shamanism and psychedelic science. Mark clearly subscribes to the conclusions and speculations of Rick Strassman in the book DMT: *The Spirit Molecule*, with his theory that DMT, also produced by the human body, is secreted in the pineal gland, right in the center of the brain—a kind of antenna or receptor that would put us in contact with other planes of reality imperceptible to the five usual senses. This would occur at critical moments in life, such as birth and death, when the organism is somehow threatened, according to the proposed explanation, or during so-called near-death experiences. Something similar would occur in the plants and animals in which the substance is found; Mark claims, for example, that black jurema concentrates more DMT in its roots during the dry periods of the caatinga, the northeastern summer. "It protects the blood from oxidation," asserts the psychonaut from Fortaleza. "DMT is considered the most potent psychedelic on the face of the Earth."

A 2018 scientific review of what is known about DMT in the organism, however, showed that research is still far from drawing solid conclusions about its biosynthetic pathways, its functions, its cerebral localization, its mental benefits, and its mode of psychedelic action. The article, signed by Steven Barker,[4] lists experimental findings such as the presence of the compound in the pineal gland in minute quantities, but notes that it is still unknown how and under what circumstances it is produced there, or whether it is also secreted in other areas of the brain and for what purpose. He characterizes as "speculation" the idea that endogenous DMT, by virtue of its ability to induce visions, might be involved in psychosis, creativity, imagination, dream states, religious or spiritual phenomena, and near-death experiences. He further dismisses even broader, "otherworldly" hypotheses suggesting that DMT and other psychedelics could provide philosophical explanations or evidence for many unresolved questions about extraordinary states of consciousness. Without mentioning Strassman, Barker points to several types of experiments that could shed light on such questions, such as trials involving continuous DMT infusion in animal models of brain injury and trauma to assess the compound's purported neuroprotective and neuroregenerative effects. "At present, the data arguing for the use of DMT as a therapeutic, particularly via administration, is thin," Barker concludes. On the other hand, six years later, in early 2024, some studies were already being published showing antidepressant effects of injected or inhaled DMT by laboratories in Brazil[5] and the United Kingdom,[6] for example.

Furthermore, another comprehensive review published in November 2024[7] surveys more recent studies on DMT, showing that the endogenous substance is present in the brain in greater quantities than previously thought and appears to participate in important processes such as neurogenesis in adult organisms, regulation of anti-inflammatory responses, and stress response, although neuroscience has not yet been able to formulate a comprehensive theoretical explanation for its functions. One of the peculiarities of this molecule is its ability to penetrate into neurons and act on receptors inaccessible to serotonin, a neurotransmitter with which it shares structural affinity but whose action is limited to receptors on the membrane of neural cells. Among the seven authors of the review are four Brazilians (Cristiano Chaves and Elisa Brietzke, from Queen's University in Canada, and Rafael dos Santos and Jaime Hallak, from USP in Ribeirão Preto). "DMT's potential as a widely accessible treatment is significant," the researchers conclude, "particularly given its potential to yield different treatment outcomes compared to other psychedelics, such as for neuropsychiatric disorders involving low-level inflammation."

Scientific research figures in Mark's church doctrine more as a tool than as the foundation of spiritual elevation. As anthropologist Rodrigo Grünewald notes in the preface to *The Path of a Juremeiro*, the IDMT proposes a path of spirituality centered on the Holy Spirit, aiming at *"a true encounter with the 'creator' of every source of life, of light, whether it be the 'outside sky' or the 'heaven from within'."*[8] As is common in the eclectic milieu of neo-shamanism, it is based on a perennialist philosophy, that is, the notion that in all times and all forms assumed by human religiosity, there is the same quest for transcendence, for contact with the divine, regardless of the manifestation it takes in different rituals. Thus, IDMT can claim its origin in the very roots of jurema, but relinquishes the mediumship now directly associated with it in the rituals of Jurema Sagrada, focusing instead on the powers of the *Mimosa tenuiflora* plant as revealed by established science, according to the doctrine set forth in Mark Collins's book:

> *I firmly believe that to get to know spirituality*
> *and the oceanic presence of the Divine Almighty,*
> *is not at all a question of simple faith anymore,*
> *but that of milligrams and what the dose might be.*
> *The mystic state is certainly a physical sensation,*
> *involving a distinct and specific chemical ingestion,*
> *of a very simple and most sacred alkaloid called DMT*

Mark's methodical approach also extends to molecules, both to the DMT that gives rise to mystical visions and to the inhibitors that facilitate its entry into brain tissue, thereby enabling the psychedelic effect. His idea is, as far as possible, to extract the alkaloids from the plants themselves, such as black jurema (DMT) and Syrian rue (inhibitors), to encapsulate them in precise quantities, in order to test successive doses of customized combinations of entheogen and inhibitor for each participant in his ceremonies. The problem arises with the so-called "entourage effect" of ayahuasca or daime, or even juremahuasca—beverages whose recipes vary from maker to maker, both in the proportion of plant materials and in cooking time, with no control over the quantities of psychoactive compounds in the final product. A higher proportion of inhibitor, for example, can cause more violent purges (intense vomiting and diarrhea), which Mark considers an undesirable adverse effect for religious experiences. He does not rule out even using a more specific allopathic inhibitor for DMT, moclobemide. In his self-assigned role as a neo-shaman, he feels unbound by the various preparation prescriptions and rituals advocated by ayahuasca and Jurema Sagrada religious traditions, yet still claims the identity of a juremeiro. "It's a tribute to a tradition that has been persecuted, exterminated, brutalized," he explains. "[A way to] draw attention to the jurema tradition itself." When asked whether he fears being accused of cultural or religious appropriation of these power plants, he admits that, yes, he has some concern:

> If I am appropriating anything, it is the substance. I do not appropriate the ritual; I do not perform Indigenous or Catimbó rituals. The ritual I conduct is one I developed myself, including with ayahuasca, derived from my work in the many churches I was fortunately invited to join.

Or, as he prefers, he has created his own syncretism.

Mark defends himself by stating that founding the one-person church IDMT to work with the DMT molecule identified with jurema, and not with chacruna, is intended to avoid appropriating a tradition from the Amazon rainforest. He asks for "complacency and leniency" regarding the way he has found to work with something that has never been equaled in his life "in terms of being fantastic and wonderful." In this way, he is fully aligned with the mission envisioned by Jonathan Ott for black jurema: to become the most widely used source for anyone to benefit from DMT. In short, to employ the analytical tools of contemporary science to make the connection with ancestral experiences more efficient from the perspective of urban psychonauts averse to tradition:

> *This practice is not playing Indian games,*
> *but visiting the same sources*
> *that shamans visit over the millennia*
> *when they cross the sacred bridges,*
> *because when one arrives at the same portal,*
> *no matter what the ritual was,*
> *one reaches the same horizons..*

Even before its official inauguration, after a decade in the making, the IDMT is already setting an example. More than four hundred kilometers from Fortaleza in a straight line, in the same Pium neighborhood of Parnamirim (Rio Grande do Norte) where I met the neo-shaman Paulo "Purna" de Azevedo, the Igreja Mirífica Eterna, or the Psychedelic Order of the Divine Tryptamine Molecule, is being established, an association inspired by Mark Collins's project. Its internal regulations, *The Horizons of Jurema*[9] were also written in cordel format with an English translation, but with some differences: the stanzas have eight or nine lines instead of seven, the rhymes and meter are more disciplined, the volume has 93 pages (compared to 373 in *The Path of a Juremeiro*), and the text took three weeks to write, not the three days reported by Collins. Its author, Jan Clefferson Costa de Freitas, was 31 years old in March 2023 when we met, a week after my meeting with Collins, who was then 63.

The differences do not end there. Jan is a slender young man with long hair, born in Natal and raised frequenting the beach at Tibau do Sul (Rio Grande do Norte), where his great-grandmother, grandmother, and great-aunts lived—midwives and prayer healers, knowledgeable about herbs traditionally used as remedies, including jurema. He attended a Brazilian public school, not a private boarding school in the United Kingdom. More gregarious than the Englishman's son, he founded his church in a meeting with fifteen founding members, not in solitude. Otherwise, the doctrine largely coincides with the perspective of neo-shamanic legalization learned from the leading figure of the IDMT of Ceará:

> *We need to found a church*
> *So that we can love the Divine*
> *To work with pure firmness*
> *To study in order to rise*
> *To the mystery of Mother Nature*
> *Of the universe and all that is*
> *To transform weight into lightness*
> *For health and well-being*
>
> *Juremeiros Walk in the Line*
> *In accordance with our Constitution*
> *It is essential to have a CNPJ*
> *Recognized as legislation*
> *And so everyone agrees*
> *Out of respect for the Sacred Jurema*
> *And the flora that grows along with it*
> *Whole of the law must be respected*

And the journey becomes more beautiful[10]

Jan's project to work freely and legally with the entheogen DMT was born from a long relationship with power plants. His initiation began very early, around the age of five. He would often fall ill during the São João festival (June 24th), his "astral hell" (he was born on July 1st). In the festivities of 1996, he was struck by severe stomach pains, and his grandmother and a neighbor prepared a medicinal brew with jurema and passion fruit for the boy. He fell asleep under the calming effect of the passion fruit, had dreams with visions of beings who came to help him, and thought he was in a hospital. Upon waking, he underwent a strong "cleansing" (vomiting) and never again fell ill during the festival season. "I remember the jurema well, it's etched in my memory. It didn't taste good."

His mother attended various types of religious services, including Jurema Sagrada terreiros, taking Jan with her, and the boy became accustomed to the presence of the plant in his life, even though it faded from his memory for a long time. From ages eight to twelve, he lost contact with this spiritual sphere and immersed himself in the interests of boys his age, such as surfing, skateboarding, and video games. At the end of this period of abstinence, he had his first encounter with ayahuasca and even attended ceremonies of the Rosicrucian Order. One day, while turning on the floodlights of a sports court, he suffered an electric shock that awakened everything: "The dreams came back, the voices in my head—but it wasn't psychosis," he is quick to clarify. He was treated by child psychologists and became the "weirdo in the family." At sixteen, from 2007 to 2010, he attended Pai Erivan's terreiro in Pitimbu, Natal, where the Jurema rituals became his favorites and where he came into contact with exus, guides, and orixás from Candomblé. The jurema wine served there did not contain an inhibitor, but people would incorporate entities all the same, which never happened to Jan, though he says he could communicate with enchanted beings, as if by telepathy or inspiration, always consciously. "I convey the messages that they, the masters, bring. People don't even notice."

In adolescence, he used other substances, such as LSD, MDMA and cannabis. At nineteen, he took jurema with Syrian rue on Pipa beach and had "incredible visions." Around the same time, he experimented with psilo-cybin from magic mushrooms with classmates from the Federal University of Rio Grande do Norte (UFRN), where he studied philosophy and would later pursue a master's and doctorate. But he wanted nothing to do with entheogens in a religious context; he was "too critical" for that kind of commitment. His group of friends founded the group Zaragata (uproar, subversion, rebellion, as the young man translates), dedicated to experiments they called "psychotropic drift": they would take various psychedelics and then discuss their effects in conversation circles. "What I seek, only jurema and mushrooms can take me there; LSD can't, it doesn't reach the eighth," says Jan, referring to the eighth and last of the "extraterrestrial" circuits of consciousness proposed by the psychologist and psychedelic guru Timothy Leary, reached, for example, in a near-death experience, consciousness beyond space-time, enlightenment.

At the age of 22, in 2013, Jan reconnected with ayahuasca churches and experienced a "very good connection," becoming fascinated by the diversity of attendees. The following year, he joined Santo Daime, becoming a fardado, uniformed member. Another year later, he gravitated toward the more distinctly neo-shamanic sphere, participating in "cross ceremonies" with Daime and Jurema in the homes of ayahuasca practitioners or in places such as the Centro Espiritualista Casa do Sol Nascente do Rei Malunguinho, led by the Jurema master Rômulo Angélico. He began to study Indigenous traditions and Catimbó, while also experimenting with various plants from the Northeast—suspected to provide inhibitors for jurema wine recipes—kept secret by the region's native peoples, such as wild passionfruit and manacá. The one he liked most was the fava-de-arara (*Hippocratea volubilis*).

Today, he has a particular preference for mushrooms, and recently, under the powerful psychedelic effect of psilocybin, he recalled that his grandmother used to say, "there are urupês [a Tupi word for bracket fungi] that are medicine, poison, or food, and there are urupês for prayer." Jan claims to have found and domesticated on Pipa beach a fungus with the characteristics and psychoactivity of *Psilocybe cubensis,* which he nicknamed *Psilocybe januarius*, in reference to his own first name and the effort it took to cultivate it and select larger, more potent varieties, using both greenhouse and outdoor cultivation techniques that he now teaches to friends.

In parallel, he deepened his academic studies. To complete his undergraduate degree at UFRN, he presented a thesis on philosophy in the poetry of the symbolist Augusto dos Anjos. He then began a master's program on the question of Being in contemporary metaphysics. For his doctoral dissertation, he focused on the concept of transfiguration in the works of the philosopher Friedrich Nietzsche (1844–1900) and the psychedelic painter Alex Grey (1953), who presents himself as a "mystical-visionary artist."[11] "Nietzsche [working] in immanence, Alex Grey in transcendence," Jan explains, who, in 2024, was working on editing the dissertation text *Transfigurações Psicodélicas: As metamorphoses da arte em Friedrich Nietzsche e Alex Grey* for publication by Dialética Editora.

Together with a group of friends, he founded the Igreja Mirífica Eterna on August 23, 2022, which has the arts as one of its four pillars, alongside science, philosophy, and mysticism. The fifteen founders make up the inner circle of the congregation, entitled to participate in the smaller, closed rituals; the larger ceremonies are open to non-members, such as the "participants" of Mark Collins's unipersonal church. Those wishing to join must undergo the "star ritual," receiving a seven-pointed star and a necklace to be worn with blue pants (a reference to the hue certain *Psilocybe* mushrooms take on when cut), a white shirt (the flower of the black jurema), and a violet cloak (the inner bark of the same tree)—other differences compared to the Fortaleza mother church, whose uniform consists of brown pants and a green shirt. Both churches, however, maintain the separation of men's and women's sections during their rituals, a remnant of the practice in Santo Daime ceremonies.

While awaiting the completion of the IDMT registration in Fortaleza to establish a branch in Parnamirim, Jan and his associates operated under the legal umbrella of the Centro Xamânico Fogo Sagrado de São José do Rio Preto (state of São Paulo), with authorization to prepare ayahuasca and juremahuasca in the Northeast. In the doctrinal book written by Jan, he and his fellow travelers define themselves as "post-materialists," recommend that the presence of entities in the sessions occur without incorporation, and even explain that mystical states should not be confused with mental illness:

> *It is necessary to understand a certain difference*
> *Existing between psychosis and mysticism*
> *The first appears to be like a disease*
> *The second does not do harm to the organism*
> *The psychotic seems very much like the mystic*
> *However doesn't know the subtle distinction*
> *The mystic travels to the metaphysical universe*
> *Without deviating from its direction.*

Each in their own way, people as different as Jan and Mark repeat in their own biographies what perennialism supposes to be the pilgrimage of human societies toward the same sacred foundation to anchor themselves in spiritual ground more solid than the uncertainties and injustices of life on Earth. Just as individuals wander from temple to temple on their journey, attending ceremonies in Catholic or Evangelical churches, Spiritist or Rosicrucian centers, Candomblé, Umbanda or Jurema Sagrada terreiros, Santo Daime, União do Vegetal or Barquinha, Osho or Hare Krishna, neo-shamanism opens itself to all trends and forms of religiosity.

Psychedelic Churches in the Anglophone Counterculture of the 1960s

Psychedelic churches are not a Northeastern, nor even a Brazilian invention, but rather a revival of a movement that began in the mid-twentieth century, inspired by Aldous Huxley's book *The Doors of Perception,* which, according to J. Christian Greer, was itself indebted to the enchanted theory of naturalism. From this perspective, each human mind would be a kind of receiver that locally channels consciousness emitted by a Universal Mind,[12] a notion echoed, for example, in the writings of Rick Strassman. Huxley is said to have embraced this belief as early as the 1930s, even before his discovery of the mystical effects of mescaline, as a member of the pacifist organization Brotherhood of the Common Life. Still according to Greer, Huxley established the two principles of psychedelicism: first, that humanity would take an evolutionary leap toward perfection by promoting the synthesis of science and religion; second, that consciousness-expanding drugs would be the sacrament enabling this synthesis.

There is nothing new under the Northeastern sun in Fortaleza or Natal, whose emerging psychedelic churches seem almost modest in their therapeutic-neo-shamanic aims compared to the salvific ideas of the 1930s and 1940s that captivated public figures such as anthropologist Margaret Mead, L. Ron Hubbard, founder of Scientology, and psychedelic guru Timothy Leary.[13] The latter, after being expelled from a Harvard University professorship, even published a manual in 1968 entitled *Start Your Own Religion.* One of the first psychedelic churches to emerge in the United States was the Wayfarers, a group Greer describes as an ultraconservative Protestant association in California, bringing together wealthy businessmen, high clergy, and the Hollywood elite. In the 1960s and 1970s, hundreds more would appear, with names such as the League of Spiritual Discovery, Neo-American Church, Brotherhood of Eternal Love, Discordian Society, Church of the SubGenius, Psychedelic Venus Fellowship, Church of All Worlds, and Church of the Tree of Life.

Many of these cults were already being persecuted by police in the 1960s, who saw them as countercultural fronts to legitimize psychedelics use, and would be targeted even more harshly after 1971, with the declaration of the War on Drugs by Republican President Richard Nixon. Not to mention, of course, the pioneering Native American Church—a syncretic religion with elements of Indigenous spirituality and Christianity, unconnected to this countercultural movement—founded in 1918 by peyote-using peoples, containing mescaline, but with roots in the nine-teenth century and still revered by many in contemporary neo-shamanism, as Greer notes: "These spiritual seekers believed that psychedelics deconditioned the corrupted customs, mores, and values inculcated by mainstream society, thereby allowing individuals to reinvent themselves according to high spiritual principles.." Among adherents of this utopian imagination, Native Americans and their cultures were seen as exemplary of these principles.

Four days after meeting Jan Clefferson in Rio Grande do Norte, my second Jurema pilgrimage through the Northeast took me to Campina Grande (in the neighboring state of Paraíba), to interview anthropologist Rodrigo Grünewald once again, with whom I had already spoken in Rio de Janeiro months earlier. Still at the hotel, before heading to his house, I watched a lecture by Greer in an online course on psychedelic science at the Chacruna Institute, in which the researcher presented a critical view of what is now called the Psychedelic Renaissance. The Stanford University lecturer of American Studies deplored the use of the term "renaissance," which in his view ignores the fact that the psychedelic movement never truly ceased to exist, but was merely forced underground before reemerging at the turn of the century. He is even less in agreement with the puritan proponents of a scientific messianism that discredit ancestral practices with entheogens and the countercultural and anarchic impulsiveness of the 1960s. This, even though the new psychedelic science has preserved the centrality of beatific visions and oceanic feelings as the foundation of the therapeutic effects sought in the rehabilitation of drugs such as DMT for medicine, so to speak purified of their chaotic and dark components in standardized scales to measure the intensity of psychedelic sessions.

In research instruments such as the Mystical Experience Questionnaire (MEQ), psychedelic scientists emphasize only positive elements, such as feelings of unity with the cosmos and nature, and disregard all other non-white cultures that, beyond the counterculture, have systematized and kept alive the technologies for the use of power plants. Nor did they necessarily do so for the "good," as conceived from the perspective of Western religions, since these plants are also frequently used for divinatory or enchanting purposes, in practices that the Christian viewpoint has always belittled and condemned as witchcraft, magic, or superstition.

The tryptaminic IDMT-Church of the Divine Master on Earth, founded by the solitary Mark Collins in Fortaleza, and the Eternal Mirific Church, led by Jan Clefferson and companions in Parnamirim, claim to be scientific heirs of the Jurema tradition of the Northeast in their pursuit of official state recognition for the DMT sacrament. Once they are fully legalized and begin their public activities, it will become clearer—beyond the intentions declared in bilingual chapter and verse—how deeply their roots are embedded in the ancestral religiosity of the Brazilian Northeast backlands, with its centuries of resistance to colonization and its accursed legacy, and to what extent they branch out on the recent surface of perennialism and psychedelic culture that speaks English.

Notes

1. Instituto Socioambiental, "Tapeba." Available at: <https://pib.socioa mbiental.org/pt/Povo:Tapeba>. Accessed: Dec 20, 2024.

2. From this point on, the information was collected through interviews conducted on March 12, 2023, and electronic correspondence up to February 2024.

3. *Mark Collins, The Path of a Juremeiro: A Philosopher's Path into Plant-Derived DMT Shamanism. Fortaleza*, CE: Emanuel Angelo de Rocha Fragoso, 2023. Available at: <https://mark.pro.br/wp-content/upl oads/2023/01/Livro-O-Caminho-de-um-juremeiro-21jan2023.pdf>. Accessed: Dec 20, 2024.

4. Steven Barker, " N,N -Dimethyltryptamine (DMT), an Endogenous Hallucinogen: Past, Present, and Future Research to Determine Its Role and Function." *Frontiers in Neuroscience*, v. 12, article 536, pp. 1-17, Aug 6, 2018. Available at: <https://doi.org/10.3389/fnins.2018. 00536>. Accessed: Dec 20, 2024.

5. Marcelo Falchi-Carvalho et al., "The Antidepressant Effects of Vaporized N,N -Dimethyltryptamine: A Preliminary Report in Treatment-Resistant Depression." Preprint. *medRxiv*, Jan 4, 2024. Available at: <https://doi.org/10.1101/2024.01.03.23300610>. Accessed: Dec 20, 2024.

6. Christopher Timmermann et al., "Effects of DMT on Mental Health Outcomes in Healthy Volunteers." *Scientific Reports*, v. 14, n. 1, Feb 7, 2024. Available at: <https://doi.org/10.10382Fs41598-024-53363-y>. Accessed: Dec 20, 2024.

7. Cristiano Chaves et al. "Why N,N-dimethyltryptamine matters: Unique features and therapeutic potential beyond classical psychedelics." *Frontiers in Psychiatry*, 15: 1485337. Available at: https://doi.org/10.3389/fpsyt.2024.1485337. Accessed: January 7, 2025.

8. *The Path of a Juremeiro*, p. 18.

9. Available at: https://www.academia.edu/123449637/Os_Horizontes_da_Jurema_The_Horizons_of_Jurema. Accessed: Dec. 20, 2024.
10. Jan Clefferson Costa de Freitas, *The Horizons of Jurema*, 2022. Pp. 18-9.
11. On his website, available at: www.alexgrey.com. Accessed: Dec. 20, 2024.
12. J. Christian Greer, "The Psychedelic Church Movement", in E. Asprem (Ed.), *Dictionary of Contemporary Esotericism*. Leiden: Brill, in press. p. 4. Available at: https://contern.org/wp-content/uploads/2022/10/a-psychurch-greer-v2.pdf. Accessed: Dec.8, 2025.
13. Benjamin Breen, *Tripping on Utopia: Margaret Mead, the Cold War, and the Troubled Birth of Psychedelic Science*. New York/Boston: Grand Central, 2024.

Life Lessons and Wisdom with the Ancestors of all Beings

Efforts to discredit and criminalize the enchanted realms of Jurema Sagrada and the practices of its masters have a long history, reducing them to belief, superstition, magic, delirium, degeneration, sin, or primitive animism. The Catholic priest and writer Antônio Vieira, among others, firmly followed this path as early as the seventeenth century, dismissing the possibility that Indigenous peoples could formulate a cosmology with fables comparable to the Hellenic paradise of the Elysian Fields. He recounted the existence of three villages beneath the earth (Ibirupiguaia, Inambuapixoré, and Anhamari) in the Ibiapaba mountains, between Piauí and Ceará, where the dead would go, "all living in great peace, festivities, and abundance of provisions." Since, in the priests' view, the Indigenous were endowed with "little malice," the European clergyman concluded that such an elaborate idea could only have been instilled in them by the devil.[1] Vieira, a mandatory figure in the Portuguese literary canon, was neither the first nor the last to propagate the notion that there is no genuine Indigenous thought or cosmology, turning his back on a tradition that survived five centuries of colonial domination, eventually giving rise to Catimbó and the Jurema Sagrada of the twentieth and twenty-first centuries.

I found this paradigmatic passage from Vieira in the doctoral thesis of the historian and archaeologist Guilherme de Souza Medeiros from Pernambuco. Defended in 2012 at the University of Clermont-Ferrand (France), its title translated into English is *The Ritual Use of Jurema among the Amerindians of Brazil: Repression and Survival of Indigenous Mores during the Era of European Spiritual Conquest (sixteenth–eighteenth Centuries)*. Despite the temporal focus, the work traces Indigenous history back to the rock paintings of Serra

M. Leite, *The Psychedelic Science of the Jurema Tree*, Copernicus Books, https://doi.org/10.1007/978-3-032-22705-8_8

173

da Capivara National Park, in São Raimundo Nonato (Piauí), where the researcher helped establish a campus of the Federal University of the São Francisco Valley (UNIVASF). Among thousands of figures painted on the rocks of natural shelters, he highlighted some that suggest the existence of rituals devoted to plants or trees long before the colonial period. It is not hard to imagine that among them was black jurema, given its ubiquity both in the caatinga and in Indigenous-inspired religiosity from the semi-arid region. Nevertheless, despite its significance, the Jurema cult also stands as a reverse icon of the erasure of these native peoples, treated as obstacles to progress and reduced to objects of natural history research—like flora and fauna—rather than as human groups with their own history, culture, and thought, the archaeologist denounces. For him, the significant presence of black jurema use in Brazil today challenges us and compels us to seek answers about a past still unknown to Brazilian society as a whole.[2]

Medeiros' doctoral thesis is a good example of how this erasure is gradually being reversed in academia, at least within research institutions in Brazil's Northeast. Since the 1970s, a robust body of literature has emerged there, treating Jurema Sagrada as a distinct religious phenomenon of Indigenous origin, rather than as a degeneration of Afro-Brazilian cults. However, this historian's relationship with Jurema goes beyond accounts found in documents researched in Brazil, Portugal, and France: Guilherme is also a juremeiro, and it was in this capacity that I met him again after a debate on psychedelics at UNIVASF and an interview on October 26, 2023, during a neo-shamanic ceremony at Aldeia Pena Branca, a terreiro in Petrolina where I participated in a session with juremahuasca.

His path to the Indigenous sacrament was convoluted. Raised in Recife in a Catholic family and school, for Guilherme, for a long time, Jurema was just the name of his grandfather's farm in Tracunhaém, a municipality in the rainforest coastal strip of Pernambuco. Fascinated by Catholic rituals, at fifteen he deepened his personal spiritual pursuits, turning to yoga and meditation. He joined a Catholic prayer group, was enchanted by Gregorian chant in Olinda's monasteries, and at eighteen entered the Rosicrucian Order. He considered becoming a monk, but was dissuaded by a female friend who threatened to report him to the monastery superior for an alleged pregnancy. He studied history at the Federal University of Pernambuco(UFPE) and fell in love with archaeology. In the 2000s, he was hired for a subproject of the National Inventory of Cultural References in the northern coastal area of his state. During visits to Umbanda houses and maracatu groups, he repeatedly heard references to the Jurema cult, but it was not yet then that he approached this form of religiosity—first would come his contact and fascination with Candomblé.

His girlfriend, a sociologist, was supervised by a Canadian professor who was researching the biography of Mãe Betinha, an active figure in Candomblé. The supervisor invited her to a grand party at the terreiro and said she could bring her partner, who was captivated by what he witnessed when the orixás arrived and he saw people with smiles stretching from ear to ear, as he recounted in an interview. "It shocked me. Where was the guilt?" the Catholic wondered. "It wasn't an empty joy, it was overflowing." During the meal offered to the guests, he was surprised to learn that babalorixá José Amaro, sitting beside him, was also a music professor at the UFPE. Soon converted, Guilherme set himself the goal of joining a maracatu group and parading with his orixá cord in plain sight (sometime later, he would discover that his leading orixá is Oxaguiã, the young Oxalá).

The immediate contact with the sacrament of black jurema would occur, interestingly, through an academic connection. Invited to an event in Recife by anthropologist Sandro Guimarães de Salles, one of the pioneers of the new generation of Jurema Sagrada studies in the early 2000s, he ended up visiting a terreiro where he witnessed people entering trance after drinking jurema wine, which, however, had no psychedelic chemical effect (certainly due to the absence of an inhibitor), as Guilherme confirmed for himself by ingesting the beverage. He attributed what practitioners described as "energy" to a placebo effect. But this typically rational explanation lasted only a short time, until he moved from São Raimundo Nonato to Petrolina in 2016.

At that time, the UNIVASF professor often heard from friends and colleagues, when he brought up the intriguing topic of Jurema, that he needed to meet "Jura" (Juracy Marques). He later learned that people were telling Marques the same thing: he needed to meet Guilherme. As predicted by their acquaintances, they eventually met, and Guilherme joined Alma, a neo-shamanic group from the Serra dos Morgados, where he began to regularly drink juremahuasca, that is, the tea prepared by Marques with black jurema and Syrian rue. To sum up what this experience meant, the historian refers to the title of a book he read about the mescaline of the peyote cactus: jurema was another "plant that makes the eyes marvel."

If the example of the researcher and Jurema practitioner is relevant here, it is not only because of Guilherme Medeiros's academic excellence, but because he embodies a harmonious coexistence between intellectual rigor and spiritual practices that some of his colleagues might recommend keeping secret. For journalism and its guiding principles of seeking the greatest possible objectivity by reporting diverse perspectives, this separation proves particularly problematic in covering the resurgent field of psychedelic biomedicine and the enduring social practices involving these substances. Since I began writing about psychedelics as a science journalist in 2017, I have grappled with the perplexity these drugs provoke and the meaning to ascribe to them.

In the field of psychedelic neuroscience, a controversy persists over whether it is appropriate or inadvisable for researchers to use the substances they study, which many argue is imperative for the experimenter to gain a clearer sense of the subjective experience they induce (the phenomenology, as the jargon goes). For a journalist like myself, from my very first report on the subject[3] it became clear that narrating one's own experiences under the effects of ayahuasca, MDMA, LSD, or Psilocybe mushrooms was relevant, and even essential, to convey to the reader something of what is transformative and potentially therapeutic in these drugs. However, along with these substances and in rituals, there also emerged certain emotional and spiritual experiences—spiritual, it should be noted, not religious, nor even mystical— that other reporters might prefer to leave out of the narrative, following the motto that the journalist is never part of the story, much less its protagonist. As these manifestations were inseparable from the personal psychedelic phenomenology, I once again followed my intuition to incorporate into the accounts in this book the various ways I had been affected during Jurema ceremonies, extending to the writing the record of my own affective responses during fieldwork.

Such was the case, for example, with the emotion stirred by the cafurnas sung by Thulny in the Fulni-ô village. A mysterious feeling, similar to what I experienced when receiving messages from Malunguinho and Cigana, through Alexandre L'Omi L'Odó and Joanah Flor, respectively, in a Recife terreiro. The astonished and comforting humility of not doubting the presence of the enchanted masters Zé Pelintra and Pilão Deitado in the modest room of Mestre Ciriaco in Alhandra. And, above all the disconcerting situations, the unrestrained weeping on Dona Deza's shoulder as she was possessed by the Capitão, during the luminous weekend spent with the Pankararé at the Festa do Amaro in Brejo do Burgo. These unique phenomenological experiences occurred, enigmatically, when I was not under the psychedelic effect of DMT from black jurema, since the preparation ingested on those occasions apparently lacked the inhibitor. Thus, the rationalist explanation for these raptures, attributing them to the suggestibility induced by such consciousness-altering compounds in psychonautic journeys, was ruled out.

There was something more in the air, what, for lack of a better word, the juremeiros call "energy," connecting the skeptical and atheist journalist with those people immersed in an enchanted world. Not enough for a conversion, but sufficient to shake the physicalist assumptions that lead one to try to explain everything through the interaction of molecules and bodies and to admit that the fabric of reality as we usually perceive it occasionally frays here and there, allowing some degree of mystery to seep through, especially since it often emerges in a very comforting way.

Those concrete experiences made me feel, in due proportion, in a situation comparable to that of the Canadian anthropologist Jeremy Narby among the Ashaninka: as a product of rationalism and materialism, he found it sufficient not to make his skepticism explicit to the Indigenous people when they said that a soul could leave the body, propelled after ingesting a strong dose of tobacco paste, and take up residence in a living jaguar—until he himself, under the influence of the substance, became the animal. "This feline and predatory impression [...] was so vivid that it remains with me to this day. But it took a long time before I felt able to discuss it in public," wrote the shaken ethnographer. "I did not think I had 'actually' transformed into a jaguar in any measurable way. Rather, I had an intense, body-based memory of the impression of 'being a feline.'"[4]

As Narby points out, science may have determined that nicotine plays an important role in the effects of tobacco, but it does not provide a precise idea of what happens in the body, brain, and mind of a shaman who transforms into a jaguar.[5] What, then, can be said about the tears that overcame me in Dona Deza's arms? It may not have been as dramatic as feeling intensely warm, powerful, and wise like Narby-the-jaguar, but that moment with Capitão remains with me just as much, as a source of strength and courage, even without the phantasmagoric action of a substance on the body, brain, and consciousness. It all comes down to the warm contact with the matriarch, her words, and her faith—something I could only dismiss as "belief" with great epistemological discomfort, after being affected by her and her faith both physically and spiritually. To deny that lived reality, in those transporting moments at the Festa do Amaro, in the terreiro in Recife, or in the little house in Alhandra, would be an act of intellectual dishonesty, as well as an obvious ethical failing toward those who welcomed me into their world without hesitation.

The least one can do, after experiencing such situations, is to reflect on what, in our own culture and worldview, prevents us from accepting at face value what we witness among traditional peoples or practitioners of religions pejoratively labeled as animist. It is not easy. The materialist conception of reality is deeply ingrained in us, with the privilege granted to natural science in our society, and even more so in the practice of science journalism.

A more humble perspective became necessary for the observer of the Jurema Sagrada when it became clear how strikingly I agreed with what I witnessed in the ceremonies I attended in the Northeast: despite poverty, arid soil, the weight of history, the harshness of the climate, religious persecution, and land injustices, communities gather in an atmosphere of peace and serenity where even the most skeptical journalist finds a place. The acceptance of finitude and helplessness is not without a certain melancholy, however. This blend of clarity and sadness can be comforting, even when experienced without the impact of psychedelics, as happens in Jurema rituals where the wine does not contain the inhibitor—and as happened to me when I broke down in tears in Dona Deza's arms.

Notes

1. *Relação da Missão da Serra de Ibiapaba* (1656). Available at: <https:// pt.wikisource.org/wiki/Descri%C3%A7%C3%A3o_da_Ibiapaba>. Accessed: 20 Dec. 2024.
2. Guilherme Medeiros, *L'Usage rituel de la Jurema chez les Amérindiens du Brésil: Répression et survie des coutumes indigènes à l'époque de la conquête spirituelle européenne (XVIeme-XVIIeme siècles)*. Madrid: Casa de Velázquez, 2011. pp. 27-8.
3. "Ecstasy e LSD podem virar remédio contra distúrbios psíquicos em breve," *Folha de S.Paulo*, 11 June 2017. Available at: <https://www1. folha.uol.com.br/ilustrissima/2017/06/1891632-o-congresso-ciencia- psicodelica-e-o-ecstasy-como-remedio.shtml>. Accessed: 20 Dec. 2024.
4. Jeremy Narby and Rafael Chanchari Pizuri, Plant Teachers: Ayahuasca, *Tobacco and the Pursuit of Knowledge*. Novato, CA: New World Library, 2021. pp. 5-6.
5. Ibid., p. 74.

Seek Truth, Act Independently, Minimize Harm

While writing this book, I was haunted by the fear that peers in science journalism and sources in the field of psychedelic research would conclude that I had succumbed to irrationalism for devoting so much time, respect, admiration, and narrative effort to esoteric practices surrounding an obscure plant from the semi-arid Northeast of Brazil. Many of them will no doubt consider irrelevant, for this field of neuroscience and its potential clinical applications, the beliefs about the powers of black jurema and other teacher plants held by the heirs of a long Indigenous resistance to colonialism in Alhandra, Águas Belas, Baía da Traição, Natal, Recife, or João Pessoa. To this possible challenging suspicion, it is worth responding that the journalistic project from which this book results was guided by a conscious effort to strictly follow the minimalist code of ethics that should guide my profession: seek truth, act independently, and minimize harm.

Starting with the last recommendation, the greatest harm a journalistic account can cause to those who granted access to their rituals arises from not taking seriously what they say and do. It would be as easy as it would be unfair to describe what was witnessed in a folkloric or pejorative manner, as primitive superstitions or remnants of an illiterate animism. Good reporters do not act this way, but even among them one may find a certain condescending attitude, which pretends to offer an objective description of what was seen and heard, yet starts from an assumption of the superiority of Western scientific knowledge over the "science of Jurema"—a set of rules, explanations, prescriptions, and songs that varies from city to city, from temple to temple, and which has never claimed to be universal or to compete with the knowledge produced in universities. More than just visiting, recording, and reporting,

M. Leite, *The Psychedelic Science of the Jurema Tree*, Copernicus Books,
https://doi.org/10.1007/978-3-032-22705-8_9

one must attempt to understand the internal logic of these manifestations, seeking to trace in history and anthropology, among other fields, the roots of what survives with difficulty in contemporary culture.

Independence, in this context, means not adopting a single perspective to make sense of what is observed. Taking Catimbó-Jurema at face value does not require anyone to become a follower of this religion or to accept as real the existence of enchanted kings, masters, caboclas and caboclos, pretas and pretos velhos (old black spirits, female or male), exus and pombajiras, but neither is it necessary to disdain those who manifest these entities in their mediumship. When invited to make an offering or drink the jurema wine, each visitor must decide whether, by refusing in the name of detachment and objectivity, they might be committing an offensive discourtesy, or even undermining the chance to access relevant information. Independence vis-à-vis devotees and priests should be matched by a similar attitude toward specialists, who often claim to know more about the religion than its own practitioners. Sometimes this is indeed the case, as with historical or geographical data devoid of accuracy in the oral transmission of doctrines and origin myths, but it makes little sense to pit one against the other, since they are discursive records of different natures, which both sides do not always recognize. It is common to hear religious leaders complain of supposed distortions introduced by researchers in academic works about their faith and, conversely, to encounter the dismissal of traditional narratives by specialists in the name of factual accuracy; it is best not to place one's foot firmly in either canoe.

It is in the gap between them that "truth" precipitates—that is, the difficulty of establishing any irrefutable knowledge in a definitive way, as common sense would wish. If this is not the case in science, it is even less so in journalism. On the other hand, this does not exempt the reporter from striving to construct a narrative as close as possible to the facts, even while acknowledging its limitations and being transparent about uncertainties and doubts. Among the many mysteries surrounding Jurema, it is not the reporter's role to decide whether the original recipe for the sacramental wine included some kind of inhibitor to confer a psychedelic effect, or whether the source of the possible inhibitor was passion fruit, manacá, or jurema itself—especially since it is more likely that, as today, there were many recipes in the past, not to mention that incorporations of entities have occurred after ingesting psychoactively inert brews, or even without them.

Readers of this book are advised to draw conclusions with the proverbial grain of skeptical doubt, certainly, but also with a drop of goodwill toward that which diverges from the fundamentals of our worldview. By the end of this exercise, one will surely come to see power plants such as black jurema, and the enchantment they exert over human animals, in a new light. Despite the sweet residue left in the spirit, the long journey of reporting, travel, and research to delve into the mysteries of Jurema left me with a profound unease, bordering on dissatisfaction. Faced with the difficulty of clarifying my thoughts beyond emotion and fine-tuning the attitude I should adopt toward what I had witnessed, I turned to the tried and true method of seeking help from those who have already devoted much reflection to the problem. I found the possible philosophical comfort, among others, in a generous book by the anthropologist Marshall Sahlins, *The New Science of the Enchanted Universe*.

Sahlins points to the dichotomy between body and soul, between the natural and the supernatural—in a word, to simplify, what is called transcendentalism—as the root of our disconnect with Indigenous peoples and their cosmologies, as well as, to some extent, the matrix of the devaluation of the Other that rationalized and supposedly justified colonialism. This is a distinction that makes no sense for Indigenous peoples immersed in immanence, for whom the invisibility of spirits is not evidence of absence in this plane of reality, but rather of their ubiquity; that is, they inhabit the same broader world in which we all circulate, as dreams and trances demonstrate from their point of view. Spirits are not in the Beyond, but everywhere.[1] Sahlins summarizes the questionable attitude of superiority held by many in established anthropology and science by recalling Jean Pouillon's well-phrased statement to challenge the pejorative notion of belief as illusion (and, by extension, of myth as synonymous with falsehood): "C'est le non-croyant qui croit que le croyant croit" (it is the nonbeliever who believes that the believer believes).

Sahlins defends the principle that immanentist thought is not mystical, superstitious, or delusional, but radically empiricist: if something is there, if it is presented to us or by us, it is because it exists, it has more than enough reality. Apparently, transcendentalism survives within materialism as a condition for preserving the dichotomy that matters most to it: the ontological distinction between what are *facts* (or data) and what is *made* by human beings (or other agents), a distinction that, moreover, erases the etymological origin of the Latin word *factum* as "made, action, feat, enterprise." In other words, there is no reason to consider as less empirical that which is not material, but only symbolic, known, or practiced, as is the case with customs, values, rituals, and myths. Sahlins cites the Swedish anthropologist Kaj Århem, for whom transcendentalism ignores cultural worlds in which subjectivity, not physicality, is the common ground of existence.

More than a respectful, dispassionate, and distanced description of others' "beliefs," as advocated by classical ethnography, Sahlins argues for the recognition that there is no inherent superiority in the transcendentalist perspective: it is merely as valid a solution as the immanentist one for dealing with the human conditions of finitude and necessity, the predicament of living under the power of supra-human forces beyond our control, shadows with which we must coexist and contend. Both immanentists and transcendentalists are confined to their own caves, and it is the ethnographer's task—as it is, I infer, the journalist's—to describe how, in different caves—that is, different cultures—people relate to shadows and beings like themselves, in their own world. Entities, enchanted beings, and deities are not mere inventions. Humans did not imagine the gods; they merely objectified, or more precisely, subjectified, the extra-human forces by which they themselves live and die: "The forces were already there. They were not imagined. They were real, empirical, life-giving and death-dealing forces. People only gave them substantive qualities that made them negotiable, or at least intelligible—consciousness, understanding, volition, and intention."[2]

Readers of the Brazilian anthropologist Eduardo Viveiros de Castro will recognize here the parallel with his concept of perspectivism, the critique of what he calls the epistemological game of objectification in his book *A Inconstância da Alma Selvagem*, the tendency to treat the Other as a thing and not as a person, a condition that shamanic thought attributes to all living beings, especially animals. Sahlins, in fact, cites Viveiros de Castro as one of the few thinkers dedicated to a reverse anthropology that takes seriously the cultural and intellectual practices of other peoples, which implies de-substantializing our own. Without this, it becomes impossible to understand, on its own terms, a cosmology in which all living beings are human, live in society, and in which the original condition common to both humans and animals is not animality, but humanity. However, they see each other through the universal prism of the predator-prey relationship: jaguars see humans as fish, just as fish see humans as jaguars. Shamans are those special beings who can change skins and visit the (natural) foreign societies that may affect our survival, as in the case of epidemics and famines. Although perspectivist theory refers mainly to societies of animal-humans, Viveiros de Castro notes in a footnote that in the cultures of western Amazonia, especially those that use hallucinogens, the personification of plants seems to be as prominent as that of animals. It can be added that the same is observed in the Amerindian cosmologies of the semi-arid Northeast, where jurema, jatobá, angico, and other trees are also imbued with some kind of agency, with "spirit," as teacher plants, as they are called.

A particularly relevant component of Viveiros de Castro's thought for this book is his concept that these worldviews, aside from not being errors or mystifications, are vehicles of a historical self-determination that traditional anthropology denies them, for example by formulating the usual division between pure and acculturated societies, in which the former would be mechanical updates of timeless structural principles, and the latter, the inexorable result of external determinations. The anthropologist rejects this form of victimization of present-day Indigenous populations which, by labeling them as acculturated (read: degenerate), can lead to the absurd conclusion that contemporary societies, not being representative of the original plenitude, are disposable, that is, they can be assimilated into the national society without major losses for humanity. Now, if this applies to the remaining ethnic groups of the Amazon, with their obviously Amerindian biotypes, naked bodies adorned with dyes, feathers, and fibers, living in communal houses and occupying the Western imagination as ideal types of Indianness, imagine the magnitude of the threat that this concept of acculturation still poses today for the mixed-race Indigenous peoples of the Northeast, who have lost most of their languages and struggle to reinvent rituals by the grace of Jurema. There will be no shortage of journalists to reproduce prejudices, from the heights of their objectivity and detachment, as they describe with the least empathy those simple ceremonies in which mixed-race people in flip-flops strive to reclaim their share of land and dignity. But it is also possible, and necessary, to move in the opposite direction.

Why Our Mysticism and Metaphysics Are Not Superior to Those of Others

The humanities, and anthropology in particular, offer sound reasons and points of support for critically examining the natural-physicalist paradigm underlying biomedicine, which serves as a platform to eject from the orbit of science anything that, from its perspective, can be disqualified as supernatural. The same is true for most psychedelic research in its resurgence, which generally dismisses any contribution that immanentist worldviews of traditional populations have made or could make to the knowledge of power plants and their technologies of use. There is, however, an additional and decisive reason, from the perspective adopted in this book, to take with a grain of salt the detachment and uprootedness that every natural scientist claims as the guiding principles of their studies: psychedelic science itself does not strictly follow the standards it uses to demote to the status of "belief" any other explanations for the phenomenology of experiences under the influence of DMT, psilocybin, or mescaline, to name three plant-derived consciousness modifiers. Mysticism, as will be seen, remains a hallmark of much of the high-impact research published as the purest manifestations of scientific rigor.

Johns Hopkins University, a temple of evidence-based biomedicine and home to one of the world's most productive psychedelic research groups, became the stage for a fratricidal (or perhaps more accurately, parricidal) dispute between its leading researchers, Roland Griffiths and Matthew Johnson. Griffiths, who died in October 2023 at the age of 77, led psilocybin studies in the early twenty-first century that resulted in the creation of the Center for Psychedelic and Consciousness Research, with an initial endowment of 15 million dollars. The article that would make Griffiths a psychedelic hero was published in 2006 under the title "Psilocybin can occasion mystical-type experiences having substantial and sustained personal meaning and spiritual significance."[3] It was cited by 2510 other researchers up to December 2025, according to Google Scholar—an enormous impact. In the following five years, the group would publish three more papers in this vein: "Mystical experience occasioned by psilocybin mediates the attribution of personal meaning and spiritual significance fourteen months later,"[4] with 1363 citations; "Mystical experiences occasioned by the hallucinogen psilocybin lead to increases in the personality domain of openness,"[5] with 1177 mentions; and "Mystical-type experiences occasioned by psilocybin: immediate and persisting dose-related effects,"[6] cited by another 1205 specialists. Even though he was listed as an author on three of these four articles and had worked with Griffiths for two decades, Johnson filed an ethics complaint with Johns Hopkins, stating: "Dr. Griffiths has run his psychedelic studies more like a 'new-age' retreat center, for lack of a better term, than a clinical research laboratory," according to the *The New York Times* in 2024.[7]

The group led by Griffiths, despite internal disagreements over mystical practices and the spiritual convictions of its members, became known for establishing a relationship between the intensity of the mystical experience under the effect of psilocybin and the resulting therapeutic benefit.[8] This intensity is measured using the Mystical Experience Questionnaire (MEQ, in English), a psychometric instrument created in 1963 by Walter Pahnke, a pastor and psychiatrist who, together with Timothy Leary in 1962, organized the infamous Good Friday Experiment (when he administered psilocybin or placebo to two dozen theology students in Boston's Marsh Chapel). Five years later, already at the Maryland Psychiatric Research Center, Pahnke would work with William A. Richards, or Bill Richards, who is trained as a pastor and psychologist and currently works as a researcher at the Johns Hopkins psychedelic center, where he became the central figure in the dispute that would lead to Johnson's departure from the group.

As a supposedly objective tool, the MEQ questionnaire deserves attention. The original version had 43 items, later shortened to thirty, and more recently to just four questions. In the thirty-item version, now the most widely used, the statements that research subjects are asked to rate on a five-point scale include phrases such as "experience of the fusion of your personal self into a larger whole," "experience of unity with ultimate reality," and "feeling that you experienced something profoundly sacred and holy." For an instrument that claims to be neutral and universal, the first thing to note is the abstract nature of the items and the anchoring of concepts in transcendentalist assumptions, which would obviously make no sense within immanentist worldviews—in other words, a questionnaire inapplicable to Indigenous or shamanic cultures. The concept of ultimate reality, for example, as something separate from the reality in which we live, would be utterly meaningless to many Indigenous peoples.

"It is astonishing to see researchers linking positive therapeutic outcomes to mystical experience," I heard the scholar of religions J. Christian Greer from Stanford University warn in a revealing lecture during a course at the Chacruna Institute.[9] The identification was immediate with what I had been thinking about this common association of psychedelics with esotericism, something I have always been willing to tolerate in neo-shamanic ceremonies I have attended, but which irritated me when it crept into scientific articles that are supposed to provide a more solid foundation for clinical applications. Greer deplores the uncritical use of religiously toned expressions in this area of science and traces them to what he calls the "entheogenic school" in the conceptualization of psychedelics, popularized by Gordon Wasson (who introduced the Mazatec "magic" mushrooms to the West), Albert Hofmann (inventor of LSD and the synthetic route to produce psilocybin), and Jonathan Ott (apostle of DMT and juremahuasca), psychedelic heroes whose ideas are presented in previous chapters of this book.

By discarding the terms "hallucinogen" and even "psychedelic" in favor of "entheogen" (generator of the divine within), this trio subscribes to a perennialist notion of the mystical experience mediated by psychedelics. In this school of thought on religion, all human cultures would share the same core vocation for the divine, albeit covered by many layers of diverse rituals, beliefs, and doctrines—which is also, in a way, an evolutionist and ethnocentric view of religious feeling, supposedly culminating in monotheism. Psychedelic substances, in turn, would have the power to grant individuals direct contact with this supposed essence of all religions: an oceanic feeling of unity, the intuition of ultimate reality and eternal truth, the experience of the presence of a divinity common to all beings, and so on.

The alleged universality of this mystical impulse underlying altered states of consciousness would extend even beyond the human species and the history of its many religions—a reconstruction project in which perennialists seek examples of ancestral entheogens in the mysterious beverages *soma*, from the Indian tradition, and *kykeon*, used to initiate Greeks into the mysteries at the temple of Eleusis.[10] Moreover, by using these substances, at all times, humans would be doing nothing more than obeying an atavism present even in various animals, from bees and birds to deer and primates, which deliberately intoxicate themselves by ingesting plants and fungi that produce psychoactive alkaloids. With the work of American psychopharmacologist Ronald K. Siegel, the drive toward the divine that perennialists see in humans becomes even more universal, encompassing animals in intoxicating symbioses with plants: "The human pursuit of intoxication is motivated by a strong biological drive that pits individual needs against those of society."[11]

Elsewhere, Greer characterizes this complex of ideas as an ideology, *psychedelicism*.[12] In his interpretation, this way of thinking rests on two premises: 1) humanity can achieve an evolutionary leap through the synthesis of science and religion; 2) consciousness-expanding drugs would serve as the sacrament of this synthesis. With some differences, this is a starting point similar to that of the utopian thought that preceded psychedelia, whose foundations were laid by anthropologists Margaret Mead and Gregory Bateson, according to historian Benjamin Breen in the book *Tripping on Utopia*. The pair's work in the 1920s and 1930s was read by and influenced perennialist authors such as Aldous Huxley, author of *The Perennial Philosophy* (1945) and *The Doors of Perception* (1954). The problem, Greer points out, is that the theses of perennialism cannot be empirically tested, as they are based on unverifiable fables constructed a posteriori to confirm pre-existing explanations, something very common in evolutionary thinking, where the chance outcomes of blind genetic drift are converted into stages of continuous improvement toward a superior form. In this process, all the historical or cultural particularities involved in manifestations such as Asian or Amazonian shamanism are erased, forcibly fitted into the interpretive framework that casts them as primitive phases of spirituality tending toward the abstract ideal of monotheism.

The entheogenic school of Huxley, Wasson, Hofmann, and Ott does an injustice not only to the traditions of the original shamans, but also to its own, insofar as it wipes out an unbroken history of Western religious initiatives—the many psychedelic and personal churches that have never ceased to exist and are eclipsed in the narrative of the Psychedelic Renaissance. Truly empiricist history, anthropology, and sociology of the psychedelic field, Greer argues, must be agnostic, not prescriptive or normative about what constitutes a "good" psychedelic (mystical or therapeutic) experience, with research instruments biased in such a way that they leave no room to accommodate all that is negative, dark, or threatening that may surface in shamanic universes or, more prosaically, in bad trips. Psychometric scales such as the MEQ are shown to be somewhat tautological in their bias toward positive mystical experiences, which do not consider as worthy of "objective" measurement the dark emotions, terrors, and anxieties that every psychonaut encounters from time to time.

The universality claimed by perennialism finds a more attenuated, secular version in brain science, as analyzed by Nicolas Langlitz in the book *Neuropsychedelia.* According to him, a new generation of researchers emerging with the psychedelic revival left behind the countercultural impetus (blamed for summoning the conservative backlash and prohibitionism) to seek in neuropsychopharmacology the foundations of spiritual techniques aimed at a better life, a bit like the Amerindian peoples of North America found in the peyote cactus a psychedelic sacrament that gave them strength to endure ethnic differences and the hardships of colonization, gathering in the syncretism of the Native American Church (NAC). Langlitz begins by torpedoing perennialism, pointing to a clear divergence between the fear some Western psychonauts have of drugs (expectation of terrifying visions, trauma, depression) and the attitude of indigenous users (pleasant anticipation), demonstrating that cultural context significantly modulates the psychedelic experience. Drawing on ethnographic observation of life in leading psychedelic science laboratories, such as Franz Vollenweider's in Zurich and Mark Geyer's in San Diego, he notes how many of the researchers interviewed maintain varied metaphysical conceptions about the nature of the psychedelic experience and mystical phenomenology, often anchoring perennialist background conceptions in the architecture and biochemistry of the brain as shaped by Darwinian evolution, rather than in a transcendental drive toward divinity. This is what he calls *biomysticism,* which does not amount to a re-enchantment of the world, but merely attributes to biology the deep emotions pre-programmed in the brain and occasionally brought to the surface by psychedelic compounds—a way of escaping the dead end of the opposition between natural and supernatural, imbued with reverence for life itself. "The God-form was molecularized," Langlitz concludes, though he remains cautious about the mystification that still survives in a kind of intellectual parallel accounting, in which scientists segregate these convictions or assumptions into a column supposedly separate from what they operationalize at their benches and in their clinical trials. "Many of our philosophical perplexities result from the fact that concepts and practices have memories, which escape us," he warns. "We have come to put this equipment to new uses while having forgotten about its past. Eclecticism without critical history still generates a perennial philosophy of sorts."[13]

Langlitz does not, however, condemn what drives contemporary neuroscience toward psychedelics—in short, the search for a better life, mental health, and peace of mind. His *neuropsychedelia*, the concept that gives the book its title, proposes that this spiritual domain be given a secular, nonmystical character, in which science seeks to understand the restlessness of the human mind without the expectation of explaining everything, much less by recourse to other realities or any metaphysical assumptions that support them: "[N]europsychedelia is less driven by faith than by experience—by feelings not of oneness with something otherworldly but of connectedness with a material world infinitely larger than one's own finite existence.."[14] If one is to seek reference in any earlier mystical form, let it be quietism: the goal is not to achieve tranquility by obtaining what one needs, but by taking hopes and fears that afflict us less seriously, contemplating things of the world as they are, serenely, even if often accepting the impossibility of changing them.

What More Can Be Learned from the Intelligence Demonstrated by Plants

Rodrigo Grünewald recounts in the article "Sobre sereias, dragões e o que mais vier" how he chooses this or that black jurema tree to harvest roots for making juremahuasca. In the midst of the juremal, a stretch of Caatinga where these trees abound, he lets himself be guided by intuition, as if by a scent: "What drew me in? Are the plants calling, communicating? Why dismiss that?" When the brew prepared with jurema and Syrian rue is ready and he drinks the psychedelic tea, a lemon balm shrub from his garden in Campina Grande radiates blue sparks among its leaves, and this is the only plant with which he has such an experience. "Is it a projection of mine onto that plant? For me, it's not," the anthropologist states. "It's a domain of nature's communication with me. Can this be assessed by the hegemonic, scientific methodology?"

There is a flourishing field of botanical research determined to prove that, yes, experimental methods can establish that plants behave and communicate, at least among themselves, in ways far more complex than suggested by their conception as ontologically deficient organisms, lacking mobility and, supposedly, the cognition that characterizes animals. Authors such as Stefano Mancuso, Monica Gagliano, and Paco Calvo are committed to empirically demonstrating that plants, far from living in a dark limbo governed solely by programs and routines inscribed in their genes, occupy some previously unsuspected point on the continuum from sentience to consciousness, and that plants think, in their own way, even though they lack brains to do so. Others, like Michael Marder, go further and argue that this plant-thinking should serve as a model to reconfigure our own way of seeing nature and treating it as a mere object for our use.

However, the notion that plants exhibit complex and directed behaviors, rather than simply vegetating in their own immobility, is not new. In fact, this school of investigation can be traced back to Charles Darwin himself, with his agnostic meticulousness in contemplating the grandeur of life. Confined to bed for weeks with an eczema attack in 1862, less than three years after the publication of *On the Origin of Species*, the luminary of evolutionism dedicated himself to observing the growth of tendrils on cucumber plants he kept on his windowsill. Over several hours, he noticed that these filaments made progressively wider circular movements in search of support, which he called "circumnutation" (from Latin roots for circle and nodding).[15] This was followed by four months of studying tendrils and 118 pages of the monograph *The Movements and Habits of Climbing Plants*. When immobilized, Darwin became able to recognize plant movement as a *behavior* (habit), or a solution to a problem posed by the environment in interaction with their climbing nature—such as growing toward light without investing in a rigid, woody body. Plants are sessile, rooted in the soil, but not incapable of movement—we are simply incompetent at perceiving it, given the acceleration characteristic of animals endowed with locomotion to escape danger or prey on the slower. In our zoocentrism, we regard plants as inanimate beings, inert objects, and not as active subjects.

Subjects? Yes, Francis Darwin, third son of the creator of evolutionary theory and the first naturalist to assert at a scientific gathering that plants possess intelligence, would affirm this in 1908. At the annual congress of the British Association for the Advancement of Science, as reported by Stefano Mancuso, the professor of plant physiology declared unequivocally that plants were intelligent organisms, not so different from animals.[16] Paco Calvo follows Francis Darwin and Mancuso in concluding that plants are capable of integrating information from their environment and display enough flexibility to modify their own behavior to adapt to situations presented by their surroundings, even retaining memory of this—in other words, they act on the subtle threshold between adaptation and cognition.

Monica Gagliano's experiments with the habituation of sensitive plants (*Mimosa pudica*), shrubs related to black jurema that close their leaflets when disturbed, are well-known: with repeated stimulation, as in the case of shelves with pots moving up and down, the leaves eventually stop closing, a memory that lasts up to forty days. More than that: they also show some form of discernment, as they resume folding their leaflets if the support moves laterally, from left to right and vice versa, but not up and down.

The fact that science has not yet been able to establish the mechanisms, sensory organs, and information processing pathways that allow plants to behave in a, let's say, "intentional" manner does not justify concluding that they lack intelligence simply because they do not possess brains to integrate data and generate actions in a centralized way as animals do. Perhaps it is more a matter of broadening the concept of intelligence and coming to see animal and human cognition as special and particularly complex cases of a more general attribute of living beings. Calvo speaks of a neurobiology of beings without neurons, capable of predictive processing: "We need to view them, like animals, as information processors with complex algorithms that turn sensory data into representations of the outside world."[17]

For Mancuso, plant intelligence follows their modular, cooperative, and distributed architecture, without command centers, capable of withstanding catastrophic and repeated predation. The most important "organ" of the plant would be the root system, this myriad of root tips growing in all directions in the soil, simultaneously sampling the presence of water, nutrients, and other organisms—from competing plants to fungi and symbiotic or pathogenic microorganisms—information that guides both the growth of each bud and of the entire system like a kind of collective brain. In a single cubic centimeter of soil, more than a thousand rootlets have been counted, which means that millions or billions of them probe, like a shadowy swarm, the soil around a single forest tree.

Plants do even more intriguing things, exhibiting behaviors we hesitate to describe as intentional only because we tend to conceive of intentionality as an attribute exclusive to individuals with fixed anatomy, mobility, and a pre-programmed lifespan, not to beings composed of collectives of more or less autonomous parts, with a vocation to perpetuate themselves or, at least, survive from a much broader temporal perspective than that of animal specimens. This agency of plants, so to speak, becomes evident in their peculiar ability to manipulate animal behavior itself, as in the case of more than 3000 myrmecophilous plant species known since the nineteenth century—plants capable of attracting and directing, through floral nectars, ants whose massive presence provides them with a praetorian guard against predators. Ronald Siegel, in his book *Intoxication*, offers abundant examples of ecological interactions in which animals become dependent on substances produced by plants, especially alkaloids that alter their perception and cognition, such as the psychedelics mescaline, DMT, psilocybin, ergotamine, and ibogaine. The observable habit of rodents and other animals that repeatedly return to consume intoxicating fruits, leaves, or seeds may have given humans clues about reliable ways to succumb to a presumed universal drive to become intoxicated and to blur the boundaries between objects of the external world and those that inhabit the dreaming, daydreaming, delirious, or traveling mind.

This more flexible view of plants as beings endowed with agency, even if not with consciousness as we know it, recognizes a dignity of their own that is gradually modifying their status in the medieval *Scala Naturae*, the great chain of beings with God at the apex, descending through angels, humans, animals, plants, and minerals. Just as, since modernity, humans have distanced themselves from angelic beings to better accommodate themselves among animals, today plants are beginning to be seen less as members of a caste comparable to inanimate beings and more as part of an expanded class of living beings freed from the yoke of transcendentalism. Philosopher Michael Marder exemplifies this categorical migration by citing the consensus on plants reached by the Swiss Federal Ethics Committee on Non-Human Biotechnology in 2008, according to which plant life not only deserves to be treated with the kind of dignity accorded to all living beings but also possesses absolute moral value.

Marder seeks in plant intelligence the seeds of a post-transcendentalist thought, insofar as he conceives of them as the invasive weeds of metaphysics, devalued, unwanted in its carefully tended garden, and yet growing in between the classical categories of thing, animal, and human. Just as Immanuel Kant grounded the edifice of pure reason in the forms of perception, Marder finds at the basis of plant behavior a kind of zero degree of vitality for all beings, that existence we call, not by chance, "vegetative state" (for example, when a person remains in a coma or unconscious, but alive), and which therefore constitutes a precondition for thought itself—a proto-thought, so to speak, though the author does not use this term. Not exactly the thought of an individual, but something like a relatively disorganized collective, which makes the plant display a certain indifference to having its parts consumed by other beings, with whom it shares what is the most essential capacities in the living world: nutrition and reproduction. Plants are prey par excellence, generally incapable of preying on anything (carnivorous plants being the exception that proves the rule). In a bold conceptual move, Marder describes the plant disposition as generosity and hospitality, in its structural denial of the subject-object dichotomy and, consequently, of all domination—something from which we have lessons to learn, both for sociality and for philosophy and ecology.

What Marder calls "plant-thinking" differs from what we understand as thought because plants remain literally and figuratively rooted in the dark soil, unable to decide where to go, which is why we have developed a blindness toward them, relegating them to the realm of inanimate things because they are immobile, since they do not resemble beings that only seek to move away from darkness and rise toward the light (here in the figurative sense peculiar to transcendentalism, which places spirit above matter). "The living logic of the plant quietly prevails over magnificent systems of thought," the philosopher notes in a particularly expressive passage, "like a tree that, with its roots, puts pressure upon, raises up, and finally cracks slabs of concrete that overlay its subterranean parts."[18] As a liminal being, the plant mediates between earth and sky, between shadow and light, extracting from the soil the nutrients it uses to grow, reproduce, and nourish the food chain of animals that move across the surface.

This liminal existence, or what might be called non-unidirectional intentionality, suggests that an alternative mode of thinking must diverge from both crude empiricism and the excesses metaphysical, Marder argues. Transcendentalism fails by ignoring everything rooted in the dead and dark matter of the mind, such as the unconscious and the ever-lurking specters of hunger, predation, abandonment, and death—something akin to the shadowy basement of the soul glimpsed by me after the second dose of DMT inhaled during the experiment at the Brain Institute of the UFRN, as recounted at the beginning of this book. Something of the plant soul within us enables the blossoming of thought, the philosopher proposes. And the lesson to be drawn from this recognition would be to become more receptive to the shadowy pole of life, to reconnect with the roots of the unconscious without repudiating the light, to reshape both thought and existence as a bridge: "To become a place where the sky conspires with the earth and where light encounters, but does not dissipate, darkness."

Certainly, no one needs to convince themselves that plants think in the strict sense conceived by Marder and Calvo, as this view can easily and mistakenly be confused with crude animism. Both authors anticipate this objection and clarify that it is not a matter of anthropomorphizing plants or attributing personhood to them, but of reconfiguring our way of regarding them and beginning to respect them as beings worthy of existence, consuming them, when necessary, not as voracious predators but with the moderation of civilized commensals. In my view, no one will lose anything by considering, at least metaphorically, their unusual ideas about plants. It would be no bad thing for the environment and the survival of the human species if, guided by what science has been revealing about plant behavior, we moved closer to the inclusive perspective that Indigenous peoples have regarding them and all living beings. From the standpoint of knowledge, Jeremy Narby recommends, it would be desirable for us to become epistemologically bilingual:

> I think the key to integrating two different ways of knowing [shamanic and scientific] is to go back and forth between the two often enough and over a long period of time. Practice makes perfect. And though this takes work and dedication, I tell myself that bilinguals have more fun...[19]

The same can be said of Jurema practitioners and psychonauts in general, who speak a language so different from our Cartesian idiom, even without adhering to their most fantastic beliefs—as I have tried to bear witness with this book.

Spinoza Without God: How to Naturalize Spirituality with Psychedelics

In April 2019, I participated as a research volunteer in a study on the effects of LSD on cognition and I vividly remember the irritation of having to answer, under the influence of the psychedelic, a barrage of psychometric questionnaires. One of them proved particularly exasperating: the Metaphysical Experience Questionnaire (MEQ). Not that I knew its name at the time, but even in that altered state I could discern the clear purpose of framing the lysergic journey in a religious, or nearly religious, context—a purpose embedded in those three dozen items such as "Experience of the fusion of your personal self into a larger whole," "experience of unity with ultimate reality," and "feeling that you experienced something profoundly sacred and holy." For a stubborn atheist, such a repertoire was annoyingly far from sufficient to encompass the experiences of that memorable day.[20] It was also deeply disappointing to be immediately excluded from an online survey by Johns Hopkins University on belief changes resulting from psychedelic experiences as soon as I answered "no" to the first question about having undergone any profound change in metaphysical convictions.[21] Atheist psychonauts who had not ceased to be so were clearly of no interest to the psychedelic research revived from the ashes.

Even if there is no reason to doubt the intellectual honesty of a reference center such as Johns Hopkins, it was and remains certain that a crucial question persists for the science journalist who ventures into the enchanted realm of Jurema, among other domains of the psychedelic universe: what to do and what to think about the visions, presences, and profound emotions experienced under the influence of consciousness-altering substances, or even without them, when participating in Jurema rituals. It would be dishonest to remain silent about such experiences or to keep them in a separate ledger, given their central role both in the psychological benefits obtained at the individual level and in the motivation to write about the subject—precisely the therapeutic potential rediscovered by biomedical research. It is imperative to decide: either the visions, presences, and emotions are part of a reality independent of the tripping subject, or they are not, being reduced to fictions produced by a mind disturbed by chemical compounds, what is pejoratively called hallucinations.

Since from the outset I resisted to take them as manifestations of other realities, of supernatural entities, or of the divine, the noetic quality of these representations—that is, the hyper-real sensation that accompanies them—demanded some explanation grounded in the fundamental scientific assumption that the natural world is the only reality that exists. Not as an unprovable and unfalsifiable claim about Being, whether God or any other figure of a universal consciousness, but as a procedural rule for investigating the structure of the world—a crucial distinction for guiding science and journalism that the philosopher Chris Letheby draws between the concepts of metaphysical naturalism and methodological naturalism.[22] Since it is impossible to prove whether other realities exist or not, we are left with conducting scientific research and reporting based on the provisional premise that the reality perceived before us is the only one amenable to measurement and rational inquiry (bracketing, in the name of scientific method and not out of metaphysical arrogance, the possibility that other approaches may exist).

At the heart of the concerns of the University of Western Australia philosopher is the "comforting illusion objection" raised against psychedelic-assisted psychotherapy: it would be illegitimate and unethical to use drugs that produce delusions and supernatural hallucinations to alleviate mental disorders, because medicine would at the same time be leading the patient into error, deceiving them about reality. Letheby counters this objection by pointing out the falsity of the premise that the therapeutic mechanism par excellence lies in the mystical experience, that is, in the induction or strengthening of non-naturalistic metaphysical beliefs. This is merely the framework within which some people (and, unfortunately, some researchers) tend to interpret these paradoxical experiences, in which the individual is overtaken by an oceanic feeling of unity accompanied by a flow of images and emotions that seem to originate elsewhere. Another way to view the issue would suggest that this results solely from the so-called dissolution of the ego, the relaxation of networks and patterns of brain—or, if you prefer, mind—functioning, induced by substances such as DMT from black jurema. Not every psychedelic experience is integrated into the psychonaut's representations as a mystical event.

The Australian thinker draws on the term *unselfing* (which could be roughly translated as "depersonalization"), coined in 1970 by another philosopher, Iris Murdoch, to refer to what neuroscientist Robin Carhart-Harris, one of the luminaries of the current "renaissance," conceptualizes as increased entropy in communication between brain regions, which becomes less rigid, or the *RElaxed Beliefs Under pSychedelics* model—or REBUS. This is a flexibilization of thought and self-perception that brings the psychonaut closer to the philosopher: "Philosophy and psychedelic experience both centrally involve exposing and scrutinizing our most fundamental, usually unexamined, beliefs about self and world, rendering our foundational assumptions opaque, visible, and therefore dubitable," says Letheby.

Psychedelics do not provide access to other realities, but to other phenomenologies. That is, to alternative ways of feeling and understanding oneself, the world, and the ways we have become accustomed to relating them. Cracks open in the crystallized ego—which neuroscience itself repeatedly denounces as illusory, along with the notion of free will—allowing new representations and interpretations to blossom or take root. To deny the empirical-phenomenological reality of this process of flexibilization, attributing to it a fundamentally mystical character that only a portion of psychonauts report, is the central error of the comforting illusion objection. After all, these are not delusions, but at most what ayahuasca users call "mirações," (visions) which no one in their right mind confuses with external reality (except in rare and pathological cases). To have one's eyes and soul flooded with wonder, awe, and gratitude at the mere existence of the world is a beneficial corollary of the psychedelic experience—a spiritual communion with nature that does not quite reach the mystical, perhaps merely the aesthetic, in the fullest sense of the word, derived as it is from that zero level of consciousness, so to speak, of pre-consciousness, which lies at the existential root of all living beings: the primal impulse to stay alive, to nourish oneself, to grow, and to perpetuate life through reproduction—giving birth, as it were.

Another psychedelic philosopher, Peter Sjöstedt-Hughes of the University of Exeter in the United Kingdom, draws on Spinoza's thought to account for the dizzying perspective opened up by psychedelics. These substances would be a privileged vehicle for accessing the *Amor Dei intellectualis*, an intuitive mode of knowledge in which one glimpses that God is nature and that there is no substantial separation between mind and matter, the dichotomy posited by Descartes. "In these exceptional insights we feel *ourselves* eternal, and in this lies our immortality," Sjöstedt-Hughes describes, "*not as a soul enduring beyond the corpse, but as a mind collapsing into eternity*, even if such eternity is fleeting."[23] For the Exeter philosopher, certain psychedelic states can be better understood through the Spinozist system, just as the Spinozist system can be intuited through certain psychedelic states. Spinoza is a monist, that is, he conceives mind and matter as attributes (expressions) of a single substance, God-Nature, which is immanent and not transcendent. Thus, the ontological and epistemological problem of the relationship between mind and matter, subject and object, culture and nature, knowledge and the thing-in-itself disappears, since there can be no interaction within what is one, just as Vesper and Venus cannot interact in the sky because they are merely two names for the same planet.

Like Letheby, Sjöstedt-Hughes is not only committed to understanding the psychedelic experience, but also to conceptualizing its phenomenological foundations in order to support, legitimize, and deepen its therapeutic use. His work has helped to dispel some of the metaphysical confusion that still plagues twenty-first-century psychedelic science, for example by proposing, in 2023, a Metaphysical Matrix Questionnaire (MMQ, in English) to help patients and therapists clarify the confused ideas we commonly have about reality, which may become even more entangled after psychedelic sessions. This is a valuable tool for putting the thinly veiled transcendental-perennialist mysticism, which underpins much clinical research, in its proper place, as reflected, as we have seen, in the ubiquitous MEQ. The MMQ, for its part, draws on the analytical knowledge accumulated over millennia about the many possible metaphysical conceptions of the world and its mode of existence. There are forty statements for respondents to agree or disagree with, grouped into major themes, such as these three sentences in the Idealism group: "Only my mind exists (solipsism)"; "The reality we perceive is a projection of our minds (idealism generally)"; "Every entity has a mind and reality appears differently to each such entity (monadic idealism)."

When interviewing Sjöstedt-Hughes about the questionnaire, I sent him my reactions to the forty items (I disagreed with the three cited above on idealism) and asked for his comments, to which he replied: "It is particularly interesting that you seem to have an emergentist belief, but with some sympathy for neutral monism."[24] By way of explanation: emergentism corresponds to the conviction that mental activity is not the same as brain activity, but emerges from it; and neutral monism implies the notion that the physical and the mental are two aspects of a single fundamental substance (in my view, matter). As a good philosopher, he did not stop there and planted a provocative seed for reflection: "I wonder whether you believe that the brain is necessary for mentality, or whether you could accept basic forms of mentality in, say, bacteria."

If it is already far from trivial to convince oneself that plants possess something like thought, extending this attribute to the basal level of microorganisms seemed a risky move in a high-stakes game, but I decided to show my hand. I replied that I would not go so far as to admit mentality in bacteria; perhaps some form of sentience. That was the term that came to mind at the time to qualify the evolutionary continuum of the capacity to feel in different organisms, as a way to circumvent the fallacious categorical separation between rational, conscious humans and the rest of living nature, which is at most intuitive and devoid of self-awareness. I had not yet read Marder, Calvo, and Mancuso, but I realize now that I was already inclined to willingly consider what they each, in their own way, conceive as plant-thinking. If cyanobacteria have chlorophyll and perform photosynthesis, perhaps they are not so evolutionarily distant from plants as we humans are from plants. The phenomenon of life manifests itself along a spectrum that varies in complexity, not in essence, among beings artificially ranked in the medieval Great Chain of Being: all have in common the production of solutions to confront their own finitude, nourishing themselves, growing, and reproducing; their differences lie solely in the metabolic, genetic, anatomical, informational, and ecological pathways they have evolved to continue living.

Returning to Sjöstedt-Hughes's Spinoza, this vital drive would correspond to what the seventeenth-century philosopher understood as *conatus*, the impulse to persevere in one's own being, which moreover serves as the sole criterion of value, that is, a point of reference for discerning what is good from what is bad, since there are no absolute values outside nature. Viewed from the perspective of the twenty-first century, it now seems unnecessary to promote the Spinozist identity between Nature and God, and legitimate to retain only the idea of an ethics that his psychedelic adherent from Exeter characterizes as merely descriptive and naturalistic, not prescriptive or transcendental. From this perspective, the final stage of virtue would correspond to mastery over the passions, that is, over the negative emotions that ultimately include the fear of death. By intuiting death as fusion with the whole and not as annihilation, *Amor Dei intellectualis* also manifests as a connection with nature, so to speak a kind of secularization of the notion of the sacred, or naturalization of spirituality, which serves well as a foundation for an ethics commensurate with the social and ecological challenges of the present, in a world grappling with emerging viruses in public health and the disease of social networks, with the errors and misjudgments of artificial intelligence, and with the galloping climate crisis.

Letheby speaks of psychedelics as tools for *moral bioenhancement*, something broader than the simple therapeutic benefit methodically investigated by biomedicine in clinical trials. When used wisely, consciousness-altering substances can contribute to an improvement of conduct inspired by the model offered by the plant-thinking described by Marder, Calvo, and Mancuso, which focuses less on the satisfaction of individual needs, desires, or ideals and more on the generic celebration of life. This was the best solution I found to the enigmas and perplexities raised by psychedelics such as DMT and by contact with the enchanted realms of Jurema that enchant northeastern Brazil: a kind of Spinozism without God to get in the way.

Notes

1. Marshall Sahlins, Frederick B. Henry Jr., *The New Science of the Enchanted Universe: An Anthropology of Most Humanity*. Princeton: Princeton University Press, 2022. p. 42.
2. *The New Science of the Enchanted Universe. An anthropology of Most Humanity*. Princeton: Princeton University Press, 2022. pp. 174-175.
3. R. R. Griffiths, W. A. Richards, U. McCann et al., "Psilocybin Can Occasion Mystical-Type Experiences Having Substantial and Sustained Personal Meaning and Spiritual Significance". *Psychopharmacology*, v. 187, pp. 268-83, 2006. Available at: <https://doi.org/10.1007/s00 213-006-0457-5>. Accessed: 20 Dec. 2024.
4. R. Griffiths, W. Richards, M. Johnson, U. McCann, and R. Jesse, "Mystical-Type Experiences Occasioned by Psilocybin Mediate the Attribution of Personal Meaning and Spiritual Significance 14 Months

Later". *Journal of Psychopharmacology*, v. 22, pp. 621-32, 2008. https://doi.org/10.1177/0269881108094300.

5. K. A. MacLean, M. W. Johnson, and R. R. Griffiths, "Mystical Experiences Occasioned by the Hallucinogen Psilocybin Lead to Increases in the Personality Domain of Openness". *Journal of Psychopharmacology*, v. 25, pp. 1453-61, 2011. Available at: <http://doi:10.1177/026988 1111420188>. Accessed: 20 Dec. 2024.

6. R. R. Griffiths, M. W. Johnson, W. A. Richards et al., "Psilocybin Occasioned Mystical-Type Experiences: Immediate and Persisting Dose-Related Effects". *Psychopharmacology*, v. 218, pp. 649-65, 2011. Available at: <https://doi.org/10.1007/s00213-011-2358-5>. Accessed: 20 Dec. 2024.

7. Brendan Borrell, "The Psychedelic Evangelist", 21 Mar. 2024. Available at: <https://www.nytimes.com/2024/03/21/health/psychedelics-roland-griffiths-johns-hopkins.html>. Accessed: 20 Dec. 2024.

8. David B. Yaden and Roland R. Griffiths, "The Subjective Effects of Psychedelics are Necessary for Their Enduring Therapeutic Effects". *ACS Pharmacology & Translational Science*, v. 4, n. 2, pp. 568-72, 2021. Available at: <https://doi.org/10.1021%2Facsptsci.0c00194>. Accessed: 20 Dec. 2024.

9. "God is in the Details: Examining the Religious Biases in Contemporary Psychedelic Research". 21 Mar. 2023.

10. Ronald K. Siegel, *Intoxication: The Universal Drive for Mind-Altering Substances*. Rochester, VT: Park Street Press, 2005. p. 70.

11. *Intoxication. The Universal drive for mind-altering substances*. Rochester, Vermont: Park Street Press, 2005. p. 15

12. J. Christian Greer, "The Psychedelic Church Movement", in E. Asprem (Ed.), *Dictionary of Contemporary Esotericism*. Leiden: Brill, 2022. pp. 1-4.

13. *Neuropsychedelia. The Revival of Hallucinogen Research since the Decade of the Brain.* Berkeley/Los Angeles: University of California Press, 2013. p. 253

14. *Neuropsychedelia. The Revival of Hallucinogen Research since the Decade of the Brain.* Berkeley/Los Angeles: University of California Press, 2013. p. 264.

15. Paco Calvo, *Planta Sapiens: Unmasking Plant Intelligence*. London: The Bridge Street Press, 2022. pp. 44-7.

16. Stefano Mancuso, *The Revolutionary Genius of Plants*. New York: Atria Books, 2018

17. Paco Calvo. *Planta Sapiens: Unmasking Plant Intelligence. Londres*: The Bridge Street Press, 2022. p. 131.

18. Michael Marder. *Plant-Thinking. A Philosophy of Vegetal Life*. Nova York: Columbia University Press, 2013. pp. 179-180

19. Jeremy Narby and Rafael Chanchari Pizuri, *Plant teachers: ayahuasca, tobacco, and the pursuit of knowledge*. Novato, CA: New World Library, 2021. p.78

20. Participation in the experiment was recounted in my book *Psiconautas: Viagens com a Ciência Psicodélica Brasileira* (Fósforo, 2021), pp. 148-53.

21. Marcelo Leite, "Ciência psicodélica se afasta do misticismo sem perder a ternura." *Folha de S.Paulo*, Nov. 16, 2020. Available at: <https://vir adapsicodelica.blogfolha.uol.com.br/2020/11/16/ciencia-psicodelica-se-afasta-do-misticismo-sem-perder-a-ternura/>. Accessed: Dec. 20, 2024.

22. Chris Letheby, *Philosophy of Psychedelics*. Oxford: Oxford University Press, 2021. p. 33.

23. Peter Sjöstedt-Hughes, "The White Sun of Substance: Spinozism and the Psychedelic Amor Dei Intellectualis ", in Christine Hauskeller and Peter Sjöstedt-Hughes (Eds.), *Philosophy and Psychedelics: Frameworks for Exceptional Experience*. London: Bloomsbury, 2022. p. 212.

24. The exchange of messages was reported in the article "Da bicicleta mística à metafísica pedestre da mudança de consciência," published on April 19, 2023, on the Virada Psicodélica blog of *Folha de S.Paulo*. Available at: <https://www1.folha.uol.com.br/blogs/virada-psicod elica/2023/04/da-bicicleta-mistica-a-metafisica-pedestre-da-mudanca-de-consciencia.shtml>. Accessed: Dec. 20, 2024.

Index